James Edwards

Mathematical Modeling of Neuroglial Communication

James Edwards

Mathematical Modeling of Neuroglial Communication

Developing a Functional Computer Based
Simulation of Intercellular and Extracellular
Communication within Glia Using Mathematical
Techniques

VDM Verlag Dr. Müller

Imprint

Bibliographic information by the German National Library: The German National Library lists this publication at the German National Bibliography; detailed bibliographic information is available on the Internet at http://dnb.d-nb.de.

Cover image: www.purestockx.com

Publisher:
VDM Verlag Dr. Müller Aktiengesellschaft & Co. KG, Dudweiler Landstr. 125 a, 66123 Saarbrücken, Germany,
Phone +49 681 9100-698, Fax +49 681 9100-988,
Email: info@vdm-verlag.de

Produced in USA and UK by:
Lightning Source Inc., La Vergne, Tennessee, USA
Lightning Source UK Ltd., Milton Keynes, UK
BookSurge LLC, 5341 Dorchester Road, Suite 16, North Charleston, SC 29418, USA

ISBN: 978-3-639-00572-1

Contents

Acknowledgements

I would like to acknowledge the guidance and support of Bill Gibson, my supervisor, and Pearl, my wife.

Chapter 1

Introduction

Glial cells are the predominant cell type in the brain with a population at least an order of magnitude greater than that of neurons (Hatton and Parpura 2004). They are distributed throughout the brain and exist in close proximity to nearly all neurons (Peters et al. 1991). While their name derives from 'glue' it is no longer appropriate to consider glia as passive structures simply holding neurons in place. Glia are now understood to have important roles besides neuronal support, most especially a role in signal transmission. Neuroglia (glia of the central nervous system (CNS)) have been implicated as agents in such functions as modulation of neuronal activity, mediation of signalling between neurons and vascular cells, migraines, epilepsy and memory (Volterra et al. 2002). As such the subject of this book - chemical communication between glial cells - is an important yet far from unique function of this group of cells.

There are different types of glia. The most numerous neuroglial cell is the astrocyte (Savchenko et al. 2000), named for its characteristic star like appearance derived from the 25-40 processes (Butt and Ransom 1993) extending from the soma. Astrocytes, like other glial cells, are able to communicate with each other using both intercellular (gap junctional) and extracellular mechanisms (Cornell-Bell et al. 1990, Hassinger et al. 1996). The degree to which each of these mechanisms are used varies considerably with each astrocyte, especially with regard to location and subtype. There are many subtypes of astrocytes (protoplasmic, fibrous, velate, interlaminar and perivascular - see Kettenmann and Ransom (2005) for details) each differing considerably in morphology and location. Astrocytes, both of the same and of different types, will also differ in their expression of cellular characteristics, such as receptor density (e.g. Bennett et al. (2006)) and gap junction distribution. Other glial cells include oligodendrocytes (which provide the myelin sheath that insulates axons within the central nervous system), Schwann cells (which insulate axons in the peripheral nervous system) and Müller cells (which are a type of radial glia that exist in the mammalian retina). *In vivo*, glia differ in their distribution. For example within the macaque retina Müller cells have an average density of 27,000 cells per square millimetre near the fovea but only 10,000 cells per square millimetre near the optic disc (Distler et al. 1993). The many ways these cells differentiate and vary are an important factor in the size and spread of cellular communication.

Chemical cellular communication is generally used to coordinate multicellular responses to a multitude of possible events. With regards to glial cells, chemical cellular communication occurs within clusters with populations typically less than one thousand cells and often far fewer, perhaps less than one dozen (though the phenomenon of spreading depression is an exception). As previously mentioned, cellular communication may occur directly between coupled cells via gap junctions, which involves the diffusion of particular chemicals through permeable channels that couple cells, or through the extracellular space, in which a messenger chemical diffuses through the space between cells and may activate specific receptors on the cell membranes of many nearby cells.

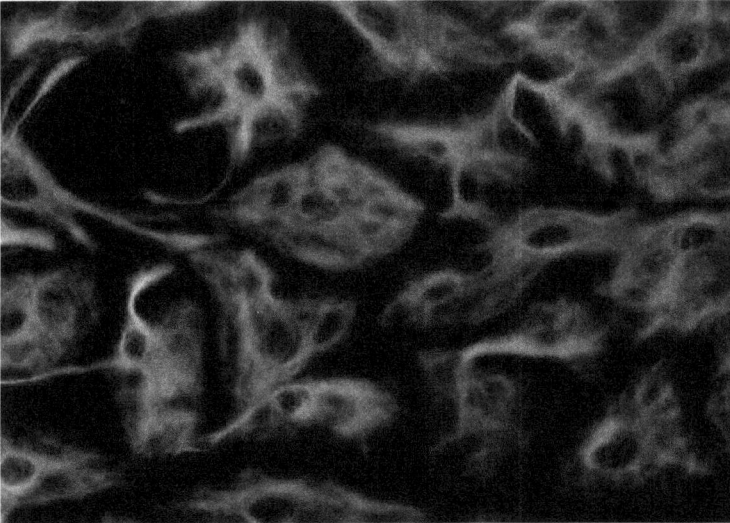

Figure 1.1: Astrocytes in culture (Armstrong 2000)

This book presents a mathematical model of chemical communication within clusters of glial cells. In the model, communication is facilitated between cells via both extracellular diffusion and intercellular gap junctions. The interaction of adenosine triphosphate (ATP), the second messenger inositol triphosphate (IP_3), ionised calcium (Ca^{2+}) and G-protein, the geometrical arrangement of cells and the heterogeneous expression of cellular traits are regarded as the basis of chemical signal propagation. The presented model is easily customisable with respect to structure, coupling strengths, receptor affinities and many other variable factors.

As part of the validation of the model, it has been used to replicate both previous theoretical works and experimental results. Simulations of the theoretical models of Sneyd et al. (1995), Höfer et al. (2002) and Bennett et al. (2005) have been compared with the present model in order to demonstrate its capacity to simulate a variety of glial wave characteristics. An experimental paper (Newman 2001) concerning glial waves in cellular clusters within the retina has also been simulated. This particular experiment was chosen as it combines a number of aspects - especially intercellular and extracellular communication - not currently expressed in mathematical models.

Chapter 2

Background

2.1 Introduction

Calcium is a universal cellular messenger involved with extensive metabolic functions. Berridge et al. (1998) called it the *life and death signal* due to its pervasive importance. Ionised calcium (Ca^{2+}) plays a large role in the regulation of many cellular functions, including muscle control, vascular operation and neural activity (Volterra et al. 2002). Most cellular calcium is protein buffered, rendering its messaging capabilities inert. A Ca^{2+} wave is a local increase in free Ca^{2+} concentration that travels within the intracellular region of one or more cells. These waves spread over clusters of cells during a time-course typically measured in the seconds or minutes (though spreading depression phenomena such as migraine may involve Ca^{2+} waves with a duration of hours (Martins-Ferreira et al. 2000)) and are believed to coordinate multicellular responses to events. Intercellular calcium waves have been observed in different cell types, such as those in the liver, in the brain, epithelia and muscle as well as glia. One use that glial cells make of calcium is as a messenger between cells and the modelling of this phenomenon is the primary aim of this book.

While the presence of astrocytes and other glial cells within the brain has been known for over a century (Ramon y Cajal 1909), the role of neuroglia in contributing to neural messaging, and particularly the study of Ca^{2+} waves within astrocytes, is only a relatively recent field of study.

Calcium waves spreading intracellularly across fresh water fish eggs were observed by Ridgway et al. (1977) and subsequently imaged by Gilkey et al. (1978). The authors proposed that calcium was propagated in an autocrine manner and that it was a common phenomenon in other invertebrate eggs. While the role of Ca^{2+} in metabolic functions had been known previously this initiated the search for Ca^{2+} waves in cells.

It was Holopainen et al. (1989) who first observed a neurotransmitter (glutamate) effecting intracellular Ca^{2+} concentration fluctuations within astrocytes. A year later Cornell-Bell et al. (1990) reported intercellular calcium waves (ICWs) between cells in astrocytic clusters. These waves were associated with the gap junctional pathway, Hassinger et al. (1996) subsequently reported the discovery of an extracellular pathway for the Ca^{2+} wave propagation after observing that astrocytes plated on a 2 dimensional substrate were still able to propagate waves between each other after the space between them had been mechanically scraped free of all connecting processes.

Guthrie et al. (1999) first identified ATP as an extracellular messenger facilitating the propagation of ICWs in astrocytes, a role identified for ATP in other cell types some years previously (for example, see Osipchuk and Cahalan (1992) with regard to leukaemia cells). Later Wang et al. (2000) imaged the spread of ATP amongst an astrocyte cluster.

Researchers such as Hassinger et al. (1996), Venance et al. (1997), Charles (1998) and Wang et al. (2000) investigated the mechanisms that initiate and mediate Ca^{2+} waves in glia. Electrical stimulation, physical agonists and a variety of neurotransmitters such as glutamate, ATP (adenosine triphosphate) and GABA (gamma-aminobutyric acid) have been implicated as factors that evoke and shape these waves.

Newman (2001) examined the contribution of each pathway in detail for the rat retina. He found that both the extracellular and intercellular pathways contributed to the spread of the Ca^{2+} wave. He also examined heterogeneous cell clusters by viewing both astrocytes and Müller cells, and how they interact in relation to the ICW. This work is reviewed in greater detail in Sec. 2.6.

Bennett et al. (2006) investigated the significance of variations in the density and affinity of purinergic receptors in astrocytes on Ca^{2+} waves, finding that it played an important role in mediating the ICW (see Sec. 2.7). In a previous study Batter et al. (1992) found heterogeneity in the amount of connexin 43, which forms gap junctions, between astrocytes in distinct regions as well as those within the same area of the brain. The effect that these types of variability have on the formation of ICWs is examined by this model.

Much of the current research in this area now focuses on neuron-glia interaction. Astrocytes are known to release the neurotransmitter glutamate (Kimelberg et al. 1990), to guide the growth of axons (Kettenmann and Ransom 2005) and to bridge the connection between otherwise disconnected neurons (Volterra and Meldolesi 2005), to name only a few roles played by astrocytes in this area.

2.2 Experimental Results

The progression of experiments developed to elucidate the underlying functions of glial cells is ongoing and is an evolving field of study. Key experiments that have been used in the construction of the present model are described in greater detail below.

2.3 Cornell-Bell Finkbeiner Cooper Smith (1990)

Cornell-Bell et al. (1990) examined the role of astrocytes in signalling and found that glutamate-sensitive ion channels responded to glutamate exposure with an elevation in their cytosolic Ca^{2+} concentrations. The authors observed that the increase in $[Ca^{2+}]$ propagated between adjacent cells, thereby forming a Ca^{2+} wave that travelled at a velocity approximately equal to that observed intracellularly ($19\mu m^{-2}s^{-2}$). This was the first paper to positively associate intercellular Ca^{2+} waves with the gap junctional pathway of astrocytes.

2.4 Hassinger Guthrie Atkinson Bennett Kater (1996)

Hassinger et al. (1996) demonstrated that astrocytes are able to propagate Ca^{2+} using extracellular mechanisms. This conclusion was reached by physically scraping cell free lanes in astrocyte cultures and elevating intracellular $[Ca^{2+}]$ by applying a electrical stimulus to a single astrocyte in the culture. It was observed that these waves could cross over the cell free lanes into distant ($\approx 120\mu m$) astrocytes. A second observation was that the distance the wave could cross to the isolated astrocyte was not dependent on the location of the stimulated astrocyte but rather was dependent on the distances between intermediate astrocytes. This indicated that not only does communication occur via an extracellular pathway, but that astrocytes can actively propagate ICWs.

Within astrocyte cultures Ca^{2+} does not itself travel extracellularly in significant quantities so the authors examined the role of the primary extracellular messenger candidate at the time, glutamate. Glutamate receptor antagonists were applied but no significant degradation in the signal was observed, indicating that glutamate is not the extracellular messenger responsible for Ca^{2+} wave propagation (at least in the astrocytes studied).

Hassinger et al. (1996) also observed equal velocities for wave propagation for both cultures of isolated and confluent astrocytes. This suggests that the wave velocity is limited by the extracellular messenger rather than any (potential) gap junctional communication. It should be noted however that astrocytes in the cortex of rat pups, on which the experiments were performed, are only weakly coupled by gap junctions (see Lee et al. (1994)). Astrocytes that are strongly coupled may not be bound by the speed of extracellular diffusion.

2.5 Wang Haydon Yeung (2000)

Extending on Guthrie et al. (1999) and Cotrina et al. (1998), the experimental results of Wang et al. (2000) provided images of agonist stimulated ATP release amongst a cluster of astrocytes.

This series of experiments also provided timed images of calcium release, a technique already well established but enabling the comparison of the concentration time-courses of ATP and Ca^{2+} waves. These experiments provided a number of significant results, the most controversial of which was that ATP release is independent of calcium. It should be noted however that other researchers, such as Coco et al. (2003), have found contradictory results that indicate that astrocytes can respond to elevations in Ca^{2+} by releasing ATP.

Wang et al. (2000) also provided information on other aspects of glial behaviour. The observation that ATP release was independent of calcium and that its wave front preceded that of Ca^{2+} suggested that ATP is a factor in calcium release itself. The different characteristics of the two chemicals - in particular that ATP is principally an extracellular messenger whereas calcium is predominantly an intracellular and intercellular messenger - implies that a direct linear relationship between the concentrations is unlikely. The results do however suggest that the wave spreads of the two chemicals are closely associated. To further explore this, part of the experiments involved the application of purinergic antagonists. This blocked both ATP (as expected) and calcium waves, indicating that calcium release requires the presence of ATP. Conversely, blocking calcium release did not impact on the spread of ATP suggesting that ATP release is independent of calcium.

Some information was garnered on the recovery of ATP and calcium by repetitive stimulation of the same astrocyte. The experiments indicated that ATP release decreases upon repeated physical stimulation such that upon a third application of stimulus within approximately one minute no ATP release is detectable. The results for calcium were very similar. It is likely that this is due to exhaustion of cellular stores and hence these results give an indication of recovery times for these chemicals in astrocytes.

A further aspect of the experiments demonstrated that ATP is an extracellular messenger, rather than an intercellular one (i.e. via gap junctions). This highlights the importance of diffusion on the wave spread, and the need to accommodate both pathways in generic models (as is done in the present model). Conversely, later research by Stout et al. (2002) has shown that ATP can be transported between astrocytes via gap junctions as well.

One further important experiment in this series demonstrated that inhibition of phospholipase C (PLCβ is a G-protein associated subtype of the PLC family of enzymes which are associated with the production of IP$_3$) results in the total inhibition of ATP and Ca^{2+}. This suggests that the intracellular and intercellular second messenger chemical IP$_3$ facilitates the release of ATP into the extracellular space and that physical stimulation of astrocytes actually initiates the G-protein cascade rather than releasing ATP from cellular stores. The cessation of ATP release when PLC is inhibited and ATP was directly applied also suggested that IP$_3$ mediates ATP production.

Wang et al. (2000) provided a rich set of information concerning the spread of chemical waves in astrocytes via the extracellular pathway. The relationship between ATP and Ca^{2+} is particularly important to modellers, a number of whom have used these results in constructing simulations of astrocytic wave spread, specifically Bennett et al. (2005), Höfer et al. (2002) and Iacobas et al.

(2006), that are described later in section Sec. 2.9.

2.6 Newman (2001)

Neuroglial cells are spread throughout the nervous system and there is often a widely divergent expression of characteristics in the astrocytes of different areas. Newman (2001) examined astrocytes and Müller cells within the rat retina in order to measure the different contributions made by both intercellular gap junctions and extracellular diffusion. The predominant glial cell in the retina, Müller cells are long, radial glia that ensheath groups of retinal neurons. They bridge neuronal and non-neuronal components of the retina, including astrocytes. These two glial cell types have considerably different characteristics, for instance in the gap junction permeability to different chemicals and the sensitivity of their receptors.

As with Wang et al. (2000), the experiments proceeded by physically simulating an astrocyte in order to produce the well known calcium wave phenomenon. A control experiment was performed and then followed by a series of experiments where various inhibitors had been applied to the culture. This enabled the contributions of the various propagation mechanisms to be identified.

Newman (2001) demonstrated that extracellular diffusion of ATP is a significant factor in the velocity and radius of a calcium wave produced within the retina. The results indicate that intercellular communication via gap junctions is also a significant factor in the characteristics of the wave, and that gap junctions are potentially capable of producing a reduced wave while purinergic receptor antagonists block extracellular messengers. Information was also provided concerning the role of astrocytes and Müller cells within the retina and how they collaborate in message transmission.

The control experiment involved mechanically stimulating a single astrocyte soma at the surface of the retina. The resulting Ca^{2+} and ATP waves were imaged and showed that the waves passed into both astrocytes and Müller cells for a radius of approximately 85μm (reached after 9.5 seconds). This equates to over one hundred Müller cells and around a dozen astrocytes (Distler et al. 1993, Distler and Dreher 1996), though the images included by Newman (2001) indicate at least six astrocytes. It should be noted that the density of glial cells varies widely within the retina.

Octanol inhibits gap junctional communication between astrocytes and Müller cells, though not between astrocytes and other astrocytes for which there is no effective inhibitor. The application of octanol resulted in a significantly increased calcium wave radius (20% increase). This surprising result was not explained by Newman, though it is possible that the octanol induced inhibition of intercellular transport of IP_3 increases the $[IP_3]$ in the central cell and thereby causes more ATP to be released from it. The release of a higher ATP concentration leads to a wider wave radius. This result suggests that the role played by gap junctional communication between astrocytes and Müller cells - glial cells of a very different character - is significant in so far as it relates to the wave spread and velocity of calcium and ATP.

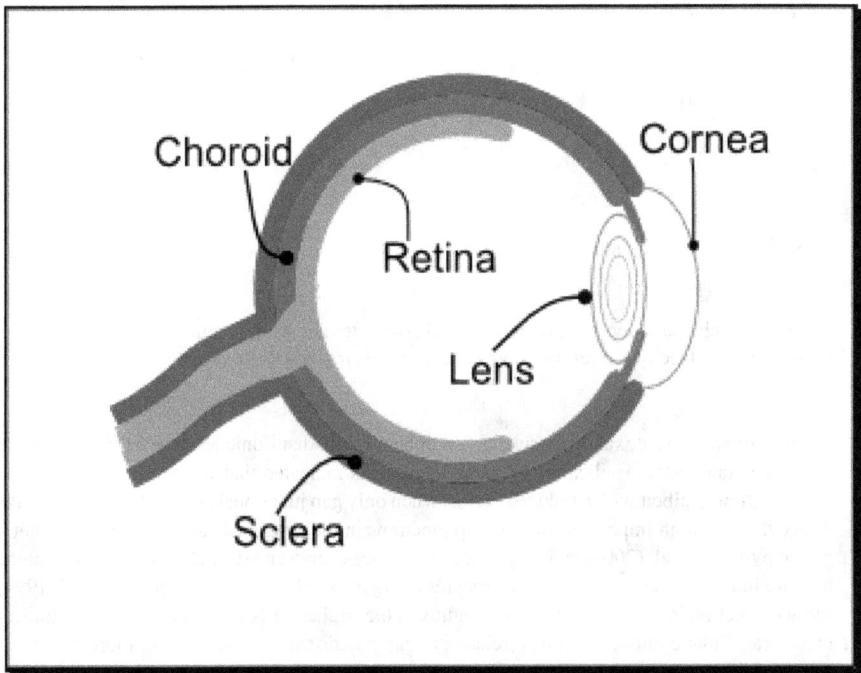

Figure 2.1: The retina is part of the central nervous system and contains both astrocytes and Müller cells. The photoreceptor cells within it receive light via the lens and the information it contains is formed into images.

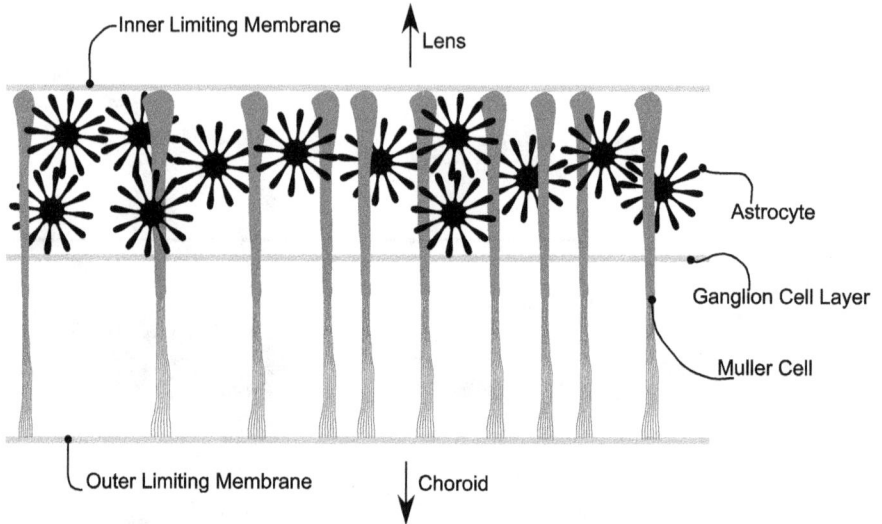

Figure 2.2: Schematic representation of retinal astrocytes and Müller cells. Astrocytes are typically found at the surface of the retina whereas Müller cells traverse the entire depth.

Suramin and pyridoxal-5-phosphate-6-azophenyl-2'4'-disulfonic acid (PPADS) are purinergic receptor antagonists. Application of these antagonists indicated that wave spread amongst astrocytes continues, albeit with a reduced radius, when only gap junctional communication is available. This evidence of an important role for gap junctions in the spread of calcium waves was not suggested by Wang et al. (2000) and may reflect differences between astrocytes in the cortex compared to those in the retina such as retinal astrocytes being relatively highly coupled (Lee et al. 1994). A further effect noticed was that the wave radius in the Müller cells was greatly reduced, indicating that extracellular communication is (relative to gap junctional communication) more significant in Müller cells than in retinal astrocytes.

Apyrase hydrolyses ATP which, as expected, gave results similar to that of suramin and PPADS. The results from application of apyrase further indicated that gap junctions are an important mechanism in calcium wave spread within retinal astrocytes and that Müller cells rely relatively more on extracellular diffusion to propagate calcium waves.

A further result obtained in these experiments was that ATP is the only extracellular messenger involved in the spread of calcium waves. In particular glutamate is not a messenger in retinal astrocytes, a result also indicated by previous experiments (Newman and Zahs 1997). This is important for the present model's construction because it means that it only requires a single extracellular messenger be included.

11

The results of Newman (2001) suggest that models of glial cells that neglect either gap junctional or extracellular communication are insufficient to describe the full range of behaviour for glial clusters, at least in the mammalian retina. Furthermore, the differences and interactions of different types of glial cells require special consideration when modelling.

2.7   Bennett Buljan Farnell Gibson (2006)

Bennett et al. (2006) grew rat spinal-astrocyte cells within narrow lanes on a 2 dimensional substrate and stimulated single astrocytes to evoke Ca^{2+} waves. This provided a means of measuring the extent and velocity of the ICWs in a structured and systematic way as it eliminates much of the structural irregularity found *in vivo*.

Preferential paths for Ca^{2+} waves (in which Ca^{2+} waves propagate along indirect paths) were observed and attributed to the differences in densities and affinities of purinergic receptors as well as in the degree of dissociation of ATP within distinct P2Y receptors. This could be demonstrated by tracking the course of a wave after stimulation, allowing sufficient time for recovery, and then stimulating the final astrocyte within the wave. It was found that the wave produced generally followed the first path (in reverse order) by activating the same astrocytes during each experiment. Furthermore, those astrocytes stimulated in only one of the two experiments tended to be clustered about the site of the initial stimulation, suggesting the difference was due to the higher concentration of ATP diffusing around the point of stimulation.

It was observed during these experiments that the purinergic receptors $P2Y_1$ and $P2Y_2$ are localised into small clusters on the cell surface. This heterogeneous distribution of receptors, together with differences in affinities, was applied to the purinergic transmission model of Bennett et al. (2005) (see Sec. 2.13) and found to explain the observed preferential pathways.

Within the experiments the Ca^{2+} waves were observed propagating for a distance of over $600\mu m$. For the first $270\mu m$ the amplitude and velocity of the wave decreased, after which time it remained constant to the edge of the preparation (another $350\mu m$), with a decreasing number of astrocytes participating in the ICW. This concentration profile is consistent with the first $270\mu m$ being dominated by the diffusion from the initial stimulus and then the wave at greater distances being propagated by the regeneration of ATP.

It was further determined that the distance that ATP will diffuse between astrocytes in sufficient concentration to propagate a Ca^{2+} wave was partially dependent on the size (and hence the populate of astrocytes within) the astrocyte lanes. The authors suggest that this is due to the increased concentration of extracellular ATP found in areas with more astrocytes leading to a greater diffused distance.

These experiments provide a useful set of data concerning extracellular wave propagation. The information provided on the preferential pathways, initial diffusion and subsequent propagation were used in formulating the presented model.

2.8 Experimental Results Summary

The experiments described in details above, together with the results provided by the existing literature discussed briefly in Sec. 2.1, provide information on many aspects of Ca^{2+} waves in glial cells that may be incorporated into theoretical models. The characteristics of waves, the types of pathways, the various interactions supported by receptors and gap junctional permeability and the variations in receptor density and affinity between different glial cell types highlight the need for a flexible model that can mimic the disparate behaviour of glia.

2.9 Theoretical Models

The progression of experiments uncovering the methods glial cells use to communicate is ongoing and while there are many observations there is significantly less known with total certainty. This situation is partly due to the differences between different astrocytes that depend on the species they originate from, the type of astrocyte, the location of the astrocyte within the CNS, the age of the subject or from the potentially wide difference in the expression of characteristics such as receptor densities between these cells, and even between neighbouring cells due to differences in gene expression. Experimentation on glial cells is also difficult due to limitations in technology: for example indicators are not available for all chemicals of interest, antagonists may inadvertently impact on multiple facets of the experiment and the difficulty inherent in experimenting on living subjects (or the limitations inherent in experimenting on sacrificed subjects). To understand the dynamics a small but diverse variety of mathematical models of glial cells and calcium waves exist in recent literature. They each have limitations in their capability to describe glial cell communication, whether due to limitations in the mathematical description of the experimental phenomena or because the models are not intended to describe the full range of experimental results produced by glia. Key models are reviewed here, with a view to demonstrating the need for such a new model as is presented here.

2.10 Sneyd Wetton Charles Sanderson (1995)

The mathematical model of Sneyd et al. (1995) defined a two dimensional grid of airway epithelial cells which, as the authors indicate, have Ca^{2+} waves that have very similar properties to those of glial cells. This grid comprises a confluent matrix of square cells (Fig. 6.1) in which all the interior cells are completely bounded by other cells. These boundaries are permeable to IP_3, a feature that mimics the gap junctions found in glia. Ca^{2+} is the other chemical simulated in this model which produces ICWs as a result of the interaction of IP_3 and Ca^{2+} using the gap junctional pathway to spread intercellularly.

The model is initiated by an increase in IP_3 within a single central cell. The IP_3 then diffuses through connected (i.e. surrounding) cells, in each case causing an increase in Ca^{2+} concentration via IP_3 receptors on intracellular stores. IP_3 itself is never regenerated in this model. The spread of the wave is thus made possible by the positive feedback of Ca^{2+} on the IP_3 receptors. These IP_3 receptors, in a set of equations previously given by Atri et al. (1993), have three binding domains. The first is high affinity and IP_3 sensitive, and rapidly releases Ca^{2+} from the cellular stores. The second is sensitive to Ca^{2+} and also high affinity, producing an autocatalytic release of Ca^{2+} in a positive feedback mechanism. The third is a low affinity Ca^{2+} binding domain that inhibits the release of Ca^{2+}. This model supports a terminating yet autocrine Ca^{2+} wave and matches experimental observations well.

Gap junctions are the only mechanism capable of supporting communication between cells in this model. This matches the experimental evidence of the authors for airway epithelial cells. The gap junctions are not modelled as separate components of the cells but rather the entire boundary shared by two cells is permeable. The actual intercellular flux is dependent on two factors: (i) a constant value signifying the permeability and (ii) the difference in concentration between the adjoining grid squares of the contiguous cells. Each interior cell is thus connected equally to four other cells in the square matrix.

The model predicts a wave that travels with a radius of four cells, reaching its maximum radius within twenty seconds and remaining visible for around one minute. There is a noticeable intercellular delay that is dependent on the intercellular flux constant, which also affects the maximum radius of the wave. The intercellular delay increases with distance from the stimulation site, presumably due to decreasing levels of the diffusing IP_3. There is also a sharp drop off in the Ca^{2+} concentration between cells in some regions and a much softer one in others. The wave speed decreases as a function of distance at an exponential rate, which since the speed is calculated based on the intracellular concentration reaching a given threshold ($0.3 \mu M$) can be understood (similarly to the delay) as being due to the decreasing concentration of the diffusing IP_3.

This model represents gap junctions as existing along the entire boundary of the cell, so they are effectively $30 \mu m$ long on each side. While this is a perfectly valid approximation for airway epithelial cells, the focus of the model, they would be inadequate for representing glial cells such as astrocytes which have disjoint soma. In addition to this, the rigidly square shape of the cells makes observations relating to the diagonal paths less realistic as cells adjoining each other on their diagonals are only connected by the bridging actions of the two cells that share common boundaries with them, making the observation about a rapid decrease in the Ca^{2+} concentration in these cells less predictive for biological behaviour. These observations of the limits of this model do not detract from its efficacy in describing the situation it was designed for, they simply highlight some limitations.

Sneyd et al. (1995) termed the mechanisms used in this model the *passive diffusion hypothesis* because the intercellular diffusion of IP_3, which is not regenerated, drives the ICWs. This model was designed to help test that hypothesis. It has been used in later years as a basis for examining other cellular actions (such as by Höfer et al. (2002)).

2.11 Höfer Venance Giaume (2002)

Höfer et al. (2002) developed a mathematical model based around the gap junction pathway for Ca^{2+} wave signals. This theoretical model includes limited aspects of the extracellular diffusion of Ca^{2+} as well as the intercellular propagation via gap junctions, though its focus was on simulating astrocytes in the rat striatum (a part of the brain associated with motor functions) in which the gap junction pathway was known to predominate. A significant development in this model is the use of a regenerative mechanism for propagating Ca^{2+} waves. Venance et al. (1997) provided the experimental data that much of this model is built on.

The model tracks the concentrations of Ca^{2+} and IP_3 within a two dimensional set of cells. The Ca^{2+} concentration is elevated in the stimulated cell. This produces a corresponding increase in IP_3 concentration for the cell via the $PLC\delta$ pathway (i.e. the process by which Ca^{2+} releases IP_3). The IP_3 diffuses intracellularly and releases Ca^{2+} from cellular stores and this Ca^{2+} in turn diffuses intracellularly and releases further IP_3 in a positive feedback cycle. Both Ca^{2+} and IP_3 also diffuse intercellularly via gap junctions which connect cells using permeable channels. Due to both the rate of diffusion and the respective permeabilities the model has IP_3 as being the primary intercellular messenger, with the gap junctions being highly impermeable to Ca^{2+}; also the rate of Ca^{2+} diffusion is too slow to propagate a wave between cells with the desired time-course.

ATP and glutamate are not included in the model and the $PLC\beta$ pathway which produces IP_3 via extracellular diffusion is treated as a constant background process rather than as a signalling pathway.

The model was used to compare the relative importance of Ca^{2+} and IP_3 gap junctional diffusion in the propagation of ICWs. The results indicated that intercellular Ca^{2+} diffusion has essentially no effect on ICWs and that IP_3 is the important messenger. When taken in conjunction with the experimental observations of Wang et al. (2000) this suggests that for astrocytes Ca^{2+} is not an important intercellular signalling messenger, though it has an important role intracellularly.

Höfer et al. (2002) explore how intercellular diffusion of IP_3 and Ca^{2+} via gap junctions gives rise to *regenerative* propagating waves Ca^{2+} waves in astrocyte clusters. Previous works (e.g. Sneyd et al. (1995, 1998)) had not included a mechanism for the release of IP_3 in non-stimulated astrocytes and hence the wave radius was limited by the diffusion of IP_3 from the stimulated astrocyte. Comparison of regenerative and non-regenerative schemes was performed using the model and indicated that regeneration via the PLCδ pathway acts as a signal amplifier, extending both the range and duration of ICWs.

The inclusion of a regenerative mechanism leads to a requirement for a mechanism to terminate the propagated wave. One simple mechanism is the technique of structuring the experiment so that smaller and smaller concentrations of IP$_3$ are transmitted to cells as a radius expands. This is a characteristic of the model and is mediated by the rate of PLCδ activity and by the gap junctional permeability of IP$_3$. The relation of these two factors in ICW propagation is tracked via the use of a diagram giving a range of values for these experimentally non-determined factors, demonstrating that there are ranges of values for which waves are infinitely regenerative, finitely regenerative and non-regenerative. The model also predicts that the spread of the ICW is more sensitive to the PLCδ rate than to the permeability rate.

The concentration of the initial stimulus was demonstrated to be a crucial factor in determining the radius of an ICW. The correlation is roughly linear and agrees with experimental data as well as reports from other modellers (Bennett et al. 2005).

One further aspect of study facilitated by the model of Höfer et al. (2002) was that of preferential pathways for ICWs. Experimental observations typically show non-symmetric waves that are generally attributed to structural characteristics of the astrocytes' arrangement and differences in the expression of cellular characteristics, such as receptor densities, on individual glial cells. The authors note however that heterogeneously distributed cells in themselves can still give rise to concentric paths, so that it appears that the individual cellular characteristics themselves are more significant in causing these events. Applications of this model indicated that variance in gap junction coupling was critical for the formation of preferential pathways whereas PLCδ activation rate was not. Other characteristics, such as astrocyte position and PLCβ variations due to heterogeneous receptor density and distributions were not studied.

Höfer et al. (2002) provided a useful model for studying aspects of Ca^{2+} waves in clusters of glial cells coupled via gap junctions. The success of this model suggests the use of extensions to it to study other aspects of Ca^{2+} waves, such as the combined effect of extracellular signals and more extensive heterogeneity in the individual cells.

2.12 Bellinger (2005)

The model by Bellinger (2005) is a general one for calcium waves that intends to build on that provided by Höfer et al. (2002) model by incorporating the extracellular diffusion of ATP and glutamate. The model does not relate directly to a particular set of experimental results but rather provides a framework for the exploration of general effects relating to calcium waves. The mathematical equations in the model are described by the author as "dramatic oversimplifications". In particular the use of discrete rather than continuous equations to replicate the extracellular diffusion itself limits the model's utility for accurately predicting the wave characteristics, such as speed and intensity.

2.13 Bennett Farnell Gibson (2005)

Bennett et al. (2005) produced a mathematical model of astrocytic ICWs focusing exclusively on extracellular diffusion transmission and disregarding gap junctional signalling. In this way their model contrasts with the model of Höfer et al. (2002), which focused on the intercellular pathway. The chemical interactions describe how extracellular ATP binds to P2Y receptors which subsequently activate intracellular G-protein. G-protein in turn releases IP_3, again intracellularly, and IP_3 then leads to the extracellular release of ATP and so this is a regenerative model. In this model $[Ca^{2+}]$ does not affect the concentrations of other chemicals within the system, it is the other chemicals that drive the ICW. This reflects the findings of Wang et al. (2000).

As suggested by the interactions described above, the model accounts for regeneration of the ICW by modelling ATP as dependent on the IP_3 concentration and Ca^{2+} as also dependent on IP_3, which in turn is dependent on ATP concentration (via the $PLC\beta$ pathway). Initialisation occurs, as usual, through stimulation of a single astrocyte which results in an increase in ATP. This ATP diffuses extracellularly forming an ATP wave front which precedes the Ca^{2+} wave front. This initial wave is equivalent to the wave in the non-regenerative models such as that of Iacobas et al. (2006). However, the initial ATP results in further ATP release from the stimulated cell over the next few seconds (or for the duration of the wave). This both maintains the concentration of ATP and Ca^{2+} in the stimulated cell for longer as well as causing a second wave front to be created in the astrocyte cluster. This second wave front is quickly subsumed by the first and acts to increase the duration and distance of the ICW.

This model is homogeneous with regard to both structure and cellular characteristics which does not support calculations concerned with determining the causes of preferential pathways. The extracellular diffusion is modelled in greater detail than is usual in that it is three dimensional (most models are two dimensional) though the astrocytes in the paper are represented as lying in a plane.

This reaction scheme diverges from previous extracellular studies of glia communication in that it makes use of the experimental results of Wang et al. (2000) in which Ca^{2+} is not a factor in the production of other chemicals. Furthermore it uses the G-protein cascade as the mechanism by which extracellular ATP facilitates the release of IP_3 and subsequently that of ATP. The actual intracellular mechanism that causes the release of ATP is unknown, though it is putatively associated with IP_3 (Salter and Hicks 1995). In recognition of this ambiguity, the second messenger that facilitates the ATP release is modelled in a generic way that would be applicable to other chemicals if necessary.

As discussed in reference to Höfer et al. (2002), a regenerative model requires a mechanism to terminate the ICW in order to conform to most experimental observations. Without such a mechanism the ATP in each cell participating in the ICW tends to increase to excessively high concentrations. Two mechanisms are implemented in this model in addition to the inherent dissipation effects of a free-boundary diffusive model. Firstly, exhaustion of the cellular store of ATP is implemented such that the available ATP is reduced as a function of the concentration released, so that around one half of the original concentration is released 10 - 20 seconds after stimulation as would be by the same concentration of IP_3 at initialisation. This linearly decreases the ATP released by equal concentrations of IP_3. While this technique simulates exhaustion of stores it equally could simulate desensitisation of the intracellular receptors responsible for ATP release. Secondly, extracellular degradation by ectonucleotidases is implemented. These mechanisms have the effect of terminating the ATP production within each cell.

The model predicts that the relationship between IP_3 and ATP is determined principally by the dissociation constant (the rate at which ATP dissociates from purinergic P2Y receptors) and is represented by K_R. This constant, as applied in the model, incorporates other aspects of the system such as the density of the receptors and the rate of G-protein activation as a result of bound P2Y receptors. As such, K_R is an effective dissociation constant. P2Y receptors are G-protein coupled purinergic receptors of which there are a number of types, most importantly for this model $P2Y_1$, for which both ATP and adenosine diphosphate (ADP) are agonists, and $P2Y_2$, for which ATP but not ADP is an agonist (see Gallagher and Salter (2003)). The predictions give (different) ranges of K_R values for both $P2Y_1$ and $P2Y_2$ receptors and state that the lower the dissociation constant the greater the Ca^{2+} concentration. When the role of K_R is evaluated along a lane of astrocytes it becomes clear that not only does a decrease in its value lead to an increase in peak concentrations, but also an increase in the wave speed. It also impacts strongly on the maximum wave radius.

With the experimental results of Hassinger et al. (1996) and Wang et al. (2000) demonstrating that extracellular signalling has an important role in astrocytic Ca^{2+} waves, it became evident that the existing theoretical models, such as Sneyd et al. (1995) and Höfer et al. (2002) which concentrate almost exclusively on the intercellular pathway, lack the ability to model an important part of *in vitro* ICW behaviour. The model of Bennett et al. (2005) was the first to model the extracellular pathway for Ca^{2+} and succeeded in demonstrating observed characteristics of ICWs and in elucidating cellular characteristics that are factors in their formation and propagation. While the model leaves open the effect on Ca^{2+} wave speed of adding gap junctional communication to extracellular diffusion as it does not have a mechanism for simulations gap junctions, the model presented in this book enables analysis of both of these pathways.

2.14 Iacobas Suadicani Spray Scemes (2006)

Iacobas et al. (2006) presented a model of ICWs in glia clusters. The model incorporates both intercellular gap junction and extracellular diffusion pathways. This model differs from most others in that it is stochastic in nature, in that the value of many parameters, as well as the physical layout of the cells and even the extracellular diffusion, is determined probabilistically. It is a non-regenerative model that incorporates many probabilistic aspects of ICWs not modelled elsewhere.

This model does not propagate ATP but rather releases it at the initial time and allows it to diffuse away. This is implemented using a single Gaussian scheme which does not support subsequent release and diffusion of more ATP. Rather, the ATP causes the intracellular release of IP_3 which in turn releases Ca^{2+}. IP_3, but not Ca^{2+}, diffuses intercellularly via gap junctions to build an ICW. Within these constraints the model is very detailed, with many parameters available to vary and tracking more chemicals than is common amongst the range of glial models. Furthermore, the authors have attempted to incorporate the variability within existing biological structure accurately by making many aspects of the model stochastic. These include the physical position of cells within a grid as well as the expression of gap junction channels and receptor density.

The model's inherent stochastic capacity to vary both the topology and individual cell characteristics, as observed *in vivo*, and to incorporate this heterogeneity in simulations contrasts with most models which assume a more homogeneous environment and rarely account for the observed variability or preferential pathways in biological experiments. The authors have not made use of this functionality to demonstrate such phenomena however.

The lack of a mechanism to support regenerative propagation is a limitation for such a recent model. The inability to generate ATP and hence continue to release IP_3 is acknowledged by the authors who state that regeneration is not necessary to account for wave spread. In some cases though regeneration has been observed experimentally *in vitro* (most recently and decisively by Bennett et al. (2006)) and hence any model that wishes to study these cases requires a regeneration mechanism.

For the reasons detailed above, it is evident that this model does not directly build on previous mathematical simulations but derives a new framework primarily from biological experiments. Whereas the stochastic features of the model make it valuable, the limitations in the range of simulations it can perform reduce the effectiveness of the model in elucidating other characteristics of ICWs.

2.15 Stamatakis Mantzaris (2006)

Stamatakis and Mantzaris (2006) present a model that represents ATP as a regenerative extracellular messenger and supports the diffusion of produced IP_3 throughout both the intra and extra cellular space. The model is homogeneous in nature, so there are no distinct cellular boundaries. Rather, both intracellular and extracellular reactions and diffusion are spread out over the entire surface. The unusual and non-physiological structure of this model impacts on the reliability of the model's predictions.

The model incorporates ATP induced release of IP_3 via P2Y purinergic receptors. Ca^{2+} is released in an autocrine manner, as well as by IP_3. Ca^{2+} also stimulates the release of IP_3, giving rise to a positive feedback cycle. ATP is regenerated by both IP_3 and Ca^{2+}. These reactions take place at every point in the system as IP_3 and ATP diffuse through out the domain without regard for cellular boundaries.

The authors present a series of bifurcations in an effort to analyse the reaction-diffusion equations. The model lends itself to this type of analysis due to its relatively simplified and homogeneous structure. While the analysis provides suggestions as to the potential effect of varying the parameters studied, due to the inherent unphysical nature of the model structure the results cannot be compared directly with experimental results.

This model provides a high degree of mathematical interpretation to the provided results. Unfortunately these theoretical observations are less valuable due to the non-biological structure of the model itself, diminishing the significance of the results.

2.16   Theoretical Results Summary

The three models most influential in construction of this book were Sneyd et al. (1995), Höfer et al. (2002) and Bennett et al. (2005). Whereas Sneyd et al. (1995) and Höfer et al. (2002) simulated gap junction function and Bennett et al. (2005) extracellular signalling, the aim of the current model is to combine these and explore systems that involve both mechanisms. The current model will enable evaluation of essentially the same problems as these two models while further facilitating the investigation of glial cell communication occurring via both intercellular and extracellular pathways. Furthermore it will extend upon the support for variability and heterogeneity supported by the model of Iacobas et al. (2006), though in a deterministic rather than stochastic manner.

Chapter 3

Mathematical Model

Glial cells are the most common cell type within the brain (Hatton and Parpura 2004). Intercellular calcium waves within these cells are associated with the mediation of neuronal activity (Perea and Araque 2005), memory (Pasti et al. 1997) and the coordination of multicellular responses to local events (Charles 1998).

Signals are propagated through networks of glia by a series of chemical messengers. The most significant of these, and the ones represented within this model, are Ca^{2+}, ATP, G-protein and IP_3. Glutamate is disregarded as its signalling role is principally within neurons, even though it is partially regulated by astrocytes (Anderson and Swanson 2000). The strength of these messenger interactions, as well as variations in the expression of cellular characteristics, determine the nature of the Ca^{2+} wave produced.

The model presented here simulates an intercellular calcium wave propagating through a two dimensional layer of heterogeneous glial cells. The glial cells support both extracellular and intercellular signalling pathways. The model provides for regenerative signalling via both of these pathways.

Two principle mechanisms are implicated in the propagation of Ca^{2+} waves throughout glial clusters: (1) gap junctions (which diffuse the IP_3 that releases Ca^{2+} in neighboring cells and are associated with $PLC\delta$) and (2) extracellular diffusion of ATP (which triggers the G-protein cascade that in turn releases intracellular Ca^{2+} and is associated with $PLC\beta$). Previous mathematical models have focused predominantly on either one of the mechanisms: gap junctions (Höfer et al. 2002, Sneyd et al. 1998, Iacobas et al. 2006) (Iacobas et al. (2006) use extracellular diffusion to *initiate* the wave) or extracellular diffusion (Bennett et al. 2005). This section presents a model that incorporates both signalling mechanisms, and allows for the analysis of how differing cell types interact using these two mechanisms.

The interactions taking place over the 2 dimensional layer of glial cells during a typical set of calculations may be summarised as:

- A cell's concentration of ATP is artificially elevated for a short duration.

- The ATP is released from the cell and diffuses within the extracellular space.

- The extracellular ATP binds to purinergic receptors on the outside cell walls of cells in the surrounding area, including the initiating cell. This initiates the G-protein cascade within the plasma membrane.

- The G-protein cascade produces IP_3 within the cell. This IP_3 diffuses and degrades intra-cellularly.

- As IP_3 diffuses it travels through intercellular gap junctions into neighbouring cells.

- IP_3 binds to intracellular receptors that release Ca^{2+}.

- The elevation in $[Ca^{2+}]$ leads to further IP_3 production. IP_3 and Ca^{2+} begin to cooperatively increase the concentration of both chemicals. A slow inhibitory Ca^{2+} binding site on the Ca^{2+} release receptor slows the initially rapid increase however.

- The raised IP_3 concentration mediates the release of ATP into the extracellular space. The ATP then diffuses throughout the surrounding space as described above.

- Internal stores of ATP and Ca^{2+} concentrations temporarily deplete as this activity occurs. This acts to suppress the continued propagation of the wave within individual cells.

- The wave of elevated chemical concentrations dissipates in each cell through a variety of effects including inhibitory activation of Ca^{2+} receptors, exhaustion of internal stores and the degradation and diffusion of chemical compounds. These effects are local to individual cells however and so the wave may be propagated to an indefinite number of neighbouring cells.

3.1 Equations

3.1.1 Receptor binding and G-protein cascade

Guanine nucleotide binding proteins, commonly called G-proteins, are a type of chemical that mediate cellular events. During the activation of G-protein guanosine diphosphate (GDP) is ex-changed for guanosine triphosphate (GTP), mediating the production of the second messenger IP_3 from the cell membrane into the cytosol.

The activation of G-protein is initiated via the G-protein cascade by the binding of extracellular ATP to the P2Y purinergic receptors on the outside of the cell membrane. The concentration of ATP, the affinity and density of the receptors and the quantity of inactive G-protein determine the ratio of activated G-protein within the cell wall.

The equation describing the current G-protein is adapted from Lemon et al. (2003). It gives the ratio of activated G-protein to the total quantity of G-protein. The derivation proceeds by defining a reaction scheme representing the activation of G-protein. The deactivation rate is constant, whereas the activation rate depends upon the current ATP concentration outside the cell membrane in the neighbourhood of the purinergic receptors (see Sec. 3.1.4 for details of the ATP concentrations):

$$G_{inactive} \underset{k_d}{\overset{k_a \rho}{\rightleftharpoons}} G_{active},$$ (3.1)

where

$$\rho = \frac{[A]}{K_R \sigma_R + [A]}.$$ (3.2)

K_R is the dissociation constant for ATP binding to the purinergic receptors and σ_R scales this value to account for effective dissociation due to receptor density. These two terms combine to form an effective dissociation value as described by Bennett et al. (2005). The cooperative model for receptor activation is used for ρ.

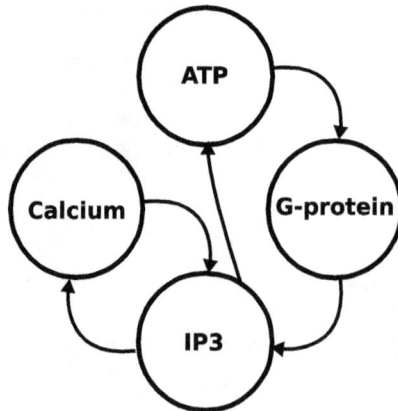

Figure 3.1: Diagrammatic representation of the interactions defined within the model. Not all interactions need necessarily apply to each set of calculations - for instance in some types of glial cells extracellular ATP diffusion is not a signalling pathway and so is not included within the calculations

Let

$$G_{total} = G_{inactive} + G_{active},$$

(3.1) can be written as:

$$\frac{\partial G_{inactive}}{\partial t} = \frac{\partial G_{total}}{\partial t} - \frac{\partial G_{active}}{\partial t} = -\frac{\partial G_{active}}{\partial t}.$$

With fast kinetics, i.e. when the speed with which G_{active} reaches equilibrium is much less than the time it takes for phosphatidylinositol bisphosphate (PIP_2) to cleave into diacylglycerol (DAG) and IP_3, this leads to:

$$\frac{\partial G_{active}}{\partial t} = k_a \rho (G_{total} - G_{active}) - k_d G_{active} = 0. \tag{3.3}$$

So

$$G_{total} - G_{active} = \frac{k_d}{k_a \rho} G_{active}.$$

Letting $G^* = \frac{G_{active}}{G_{total}}$ and $K_G = \frac{k_d}{k_a}$ we have:

$$G^* = \frac{G_{active}}{G_{total}} = \left(\frac{k_d + k_a \rho}{k_a \rho}\right)^{-1}.$$

Rearranging gives:

$$G^* = \frac{1}{K_G \rho^{-1} + 1} = \frac{\rho}{K_G + \rho}. \tag{3.4}$$

The G-protein diffuses very slowly relative to the other chemicals considered here ($\approx 1.2 \mu m^2 s^{-1}$ - $1.5 \mu m^2 s^{-1}$ (Pugh and Lamb 2000)), so for the purposes of this model G-protein diffusion can be ignored.

It is possible for G-protein to be activated in the absence of ATP, a process that has a role in maintaining the steady state concentration of IP_3. To model this requires the addition of a further term to the model, leading to:

$$G^* = \frac{\rho + \delta}{K_G + \rho + \delta}, \tag{3.5}$$

where δ is comprised of a constant value (which may be zero) and a calculation intended to approximate the necessary value for maintaining a steady state concentration. The formula for δ is:

$$\delta = \delta_c + K_G \left(\frac{G_{total} \nu_G}{\gamma_s} - 1 \right)^{-1}, \tag{3.6}$$

where δ_c is a constant and

$$\gamma_s = (k_{deg}[I]_\infty - \frac{\rho_{max}[C]_\infty^2}{[C]_\infty^2 + K_{Ca}^2}).$$

3.1.2 Intracellular IP$_3$ release

IP$_3$ is a second messenger to which some intracellular Ca^{2+} receptors are sensitive. It is formed when the G-protein cascade (PLCβ) or cytosolic [Ca^{2+}] elevations (PLCδ) mobilise PLC to hydrolyse phospholipid and produce IP$_3$.

Release mediated by PLCβ

The equation describing the PLCβ triggered IP$_3$ release resulting from the G-protein cascade is based on Bennett et al. (2005),

$$\frac{\partial[I]}{\partial t} = D_{IP_3} \nabla^2[I] + \nu_G \, G_{total} \, G^* - k_{deg}[I]. \tag{3.7}$$

The first term represents the cell wall bounded diffusion of IP$_3$. The next term governs IP$_3$ production and is only applied at the cell wall since the level of activated G-protein is insignificant elsewhere due to the slow diffusion mentioned above (Eq. 3.5). The release of IP$_3$ is determined by the total quantity of G-protein in the immediate area (G_{total}), the ratio of activated G-protein (G^*) as determined by Eq. 3.5 and the rate at which activated G-protein produces IP$_3$ (ν_G). The final term represents the degradation, which is modelled as linear.

Release mediated by PLCδ

The production of IP$_3$ by Ca^{2+} through the PLCδ pathway is described in Höfer et al. (2002) and Lemon et al. (2003). The present model takes the empirical equation provided in Höfer et al. (2002):

$$\nu_{PLC\delta} = \frac{\rho_{max}[C]^2}{K_{Ca}^2 + [C]^2}, \tag{3.8}$$

which is a Hill equation representing Ca^{2+} receptors with two binding sites and dissociation constant K_{Ca}.

Summing the contributions of the two production terms, and including linear degradation, gives the model equation for intracellular IP$_3$ release:

$$\frac{\partial[I]}{\partial t} = D_{IP_3}\nabla^2[I] + \nu_G G_{total}G^* + \nu_{PLC\delta} - k_{deg}[I]. \qquad (3.9)$$

3.1.3 Intercellular IP$_3$ diffusion via gap junctional pathways

Gap junctions are cellular structures that form an intercellular bridge between two cells. Gap junctions are composed of connexin (Cx) proteins that combine to form hemichannels (or connexons) in each cell. These hemichannels connect across the intercellular space forming a channel of $1.5nm$ diameter (Keener et al. 2001) that selectively supports electrical and chemical transmission between cells. A glial cell's gap junction may have hundreds of channels (Ransom and Ye 2005), not all of which will be open, and there may be thousands of gap junctions between two astrocytes (Rash et al. 2001). Indeed a single astrocyte may have 30,000 distinct gap junctions (Nagy and Rash 2003). These factors determine the total potential intercellular flux of a diffusing substance such as IP$_3$.

IP$_3$ diffuses relatively rapidly at $280\mu m^2 s^{-1}$ (c.f. Ca^{2+} diffusion of $20\mu m^2 s^{-1}$) and elevated Ca^{2+} levels decrease gap junction conductance (Bennett et al. 1991). The intercellular diffusion of IP$_3$ is hence modelled here as the only method of propagating the intercellular calcium wave between the cells. Other models (Höfer et al. 2002, Iacobas et al. 2006) have also disregarded the intercellular diffusion of Ca^{2+} as being relatively insignificant. Experimentalists (Leybaert et al. 1998) have likewise concluded that whereas intercellular IP$_3$ diffusion is sufficient to propagate an ICW, intercellular Ca^{2+} diffusion is not.

Within the brain, gap junctions are predominantly located between glial cells (Ransom and Ye 2005). IP$_3$ may diffuse between cells along any number of gap junctions, both homologous (between different cells of the same type) and heterologous (between cells of different types). Astrocytes tend to have distinct non-overlapping domains (Bushong et al. 2002), and so their somata are disjoint. Accordingly, within glial cell clusters, gap junctions form on the processes and this is reflected in the present model. IP$_3$ diffuses through the processes at the same rate as it does through the soma. Across the gap junction the flux is determined by the permeability to the relevant molecule, the rate of diffusion of the molecule and the difference in concentration within both hemichannels. As described in Keener et al. (2001),

$$F = P_{IP3}([I]|_{x=\xi^-} - [I]|_{x=\xi^+}). \qquad (3.10)$$

where F is the flux, $[I]|_{x=\xi^+}$ is the concentration at the hemichannel of a chosen cell and $[I]|_{x=\xi^-}$ is the concentration at hemichannel of the connected cell. The permeability P_{IP3} deter-

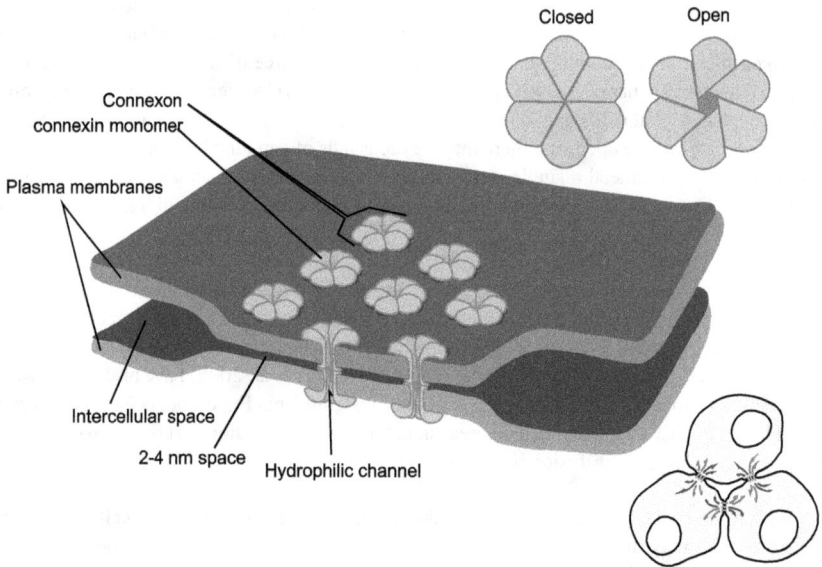

Figure 3.2: A gap junction with multiple channels. Each gap junction may have hundreds of channels, which are always composed of two hemichannels that connect two cells.

mines the rate with which the concentration changes in the chosen cell. The diffusing substance (IP_3) is conserved and so the connected cell incurs a concentration change of the same magnitude but opposite sign.

Applying Fick's law

$$F = -D\frac{\partial u}{\partial x},$$ (3.11)

to Eq. 3.10 gives

$$-D_{IP3}\frac{\partial [I]}{\partial x}\Big|_{x=\xi} = P_{IP3}([I]|_{x=\xi^-} - [I]|_{x=\xi^+})$$ (3.12)

or

$$\frac{\partial [I]}{\partial x}\Big|_{x=\xi} = -\frac{P_{IP3}}{D_{IP3}}([I]|_{x=\xi^-} - [I]|_{x=\xi^+}).$$ (3.13)

For a single cell, the total intercellular flux is given by the net contribution of Eq. 3.13 on each open gap junction on every processes that connects to another cell:

$$\frac{\partial [I]}{\partial t} = \sum_{i=1}^{\# \, cells} \sum_{j=1}^{\# \, processes} U_g(j,i)\, U_o\, P_{ip3}\frac{\partial [I]}{\partial x}\Big|_{x=\xi},$$ (3.14)

where $U_g(j,i)$ denotes the number of gap junctions with cell i on process j and U_o is the average number of open channels for each gap junction.

Applying this aggregated formula at each cell gives the total flux out of the cell, which will be negative when the [IP_3] increases. As IP_3 is conserved by this activity, any increase in [IP_3] in one cell must be balanced by an equivalent decrease in [IP_3] in the other cell.

3.1.4 ATP release into the extracellular space

ATP is an adenonucleotide affecting molecular transport, energy transfer and both intracellular and extracellular signalling. In its role as an agent of glial extracellular signalling, ATP is released from the cell wall (Queiroz et al. (1999) identified it as being released from Cx hemichannels) into the extracellular space where it diffuses. This ATP can then bind to P2 purinergic receptors, the principal type in the present model being the P2Y receptors. P2Y receptors are metabotropic, mediating intracellular $[Ca^{2+}]$ through G-protein activation (Sec. 3.1.1). Experimental results from Salter and Hicks (1995) have demonstrated that this process produces intracellular IP_3 and results in an intracellular increase of $[Ca^{2+}]$ within astrocytes.

The mechanism that triggers the release of ATP has not been positively identified, although it is putatively associated with $[IP_3]$ (Haydon 2001). This relationship implies that ATP waves may regenerate, as in elevating $[IP_3]$ by binding to the P2Y receptors they facilitate the subsequent release of ATP from Cx hemichannels.

Extracellular ATP is rapidly hydrolysed by ectoenzymes (Ziganshin et al. 1994) into ADP, adenosine monophosphate (AMP) and adenosine, to which purinergic receptors bind differentially; for example $P2Y_1$ is activated both by ATP and ADP but $P2Y_2$ is not activated by ADP (Gallagher and Salter 2003). Within the present model subtypes of receptors are not accounted for, and so the speed of degradation may be reduced in order to simulate the binding of ATP breakdown metabolites onto the P2Y receptors.

The equation used to represent ATP release, diffusion and degradation is adapted from Bennett et al. (2005) Eq. 11:

$$\frac{\partial[A]}{\partial t} = D_{ATP}\nabla^2[A] + \chi(t)\alpha_V\frac{[I] - I_{min}}{[I] + K_{rel}}$$
$$- \frac{v_{deg}[A]}{A_{deg} + [A]} + v(t, x). \tag{3.15}$$

The first term represents the diffusion of ATP throughout the extracellular space with the rate of diffusion determined by D_A.

The second term simulates IP_3 induced ATP release into the extracellular space and occurs only at the cell wall. I_{min} is the threshold level of $[IP_3]$ required for ATP release. α_V is the rate of ATP mobilisation by IP_3. The rate of release is scaled by $\chi(t)$ which represents store depletion of ATP and receptor desensitisation to IP_3 (Eq. 3.16). K_{rel} is the kinetic parameter that determines the response to the IP_3 concentration changes.

The third term models hydrolysis by ectonucleotidases of ATP, which deplete ATP at a rate determined by the respective concentrations of substrate (ATP) and catalyst (ectonucleotides). The range of values for the rate of degradation v_{deg} is large (Sec. 3.2.1) and can have a significant effect on the size of the wave radius.

The last term provides for a direct application of ATP into the system at a given point and time. This is used to initiate the calcium wave and is an analogue of the standard stimulation or bath techniques used experimentally to initiate waves.

Determination of the ATP depletion term $\chi(t)$

$\chi(t)$ simulates ATP store depletion and desensitisation of IP_3 sensitive receptors. Initially ATP stores are full and receptors maximally sensitive ($\chi(0) = 1$). $\chi(t)$ decreases in response to ATP release toward a minimum of 0 and is replenished at a constant rate (χ_{repl}).

$$\frac{\partial \chi}{\partial t} = \chi_{repl} - k_{loss}\chi(t)\frac{[I] - [I]_{min}}{K_{rel} + [I]}. \tag{3.16}$$

3.1.5 Ca^{2+} and IP_3 induced Ca^{2+} release

As described previously (Sec. 2), Ca^{2+} is a universal cellular messenger prevalent in glial cells. Ca^{2+} is released from cellular stores by IP_3 sensitive receptors within the cell. Ca^{2+} cooperatively binds to these receptors thereby further increasing the release of Ca^{2+}. Slow binding Ca^{2+} sensitive sites on the receptors later inhibit this release.

De Young and Keizer (1992) developed a comprehensive model for IP_3 dependent Ca^{2+} release in cells. This model was later simplified (Li and Rinzel 1994) to the form it is most commonly used in. The present model is based on Fink et al. (1999), modified to use differently sized pools for IP_3 and Ca^{2+} sensitive mobilisation of Ca^{2+} (Taylor and Putney 1985, Dupont et al. 1991):

$$\frac{\partial [C]}{\partial t} = \beta(J_{channel} - J_{pump} + J_{leak}), \tag{3.17}$$

where $J_{channel}$, J_{pump} and J_{leak} refer respectively to the IP_3 and Ca^{2+} induced release, pump uptake from the cytosol into the endoplasmic reticulum and the leak from the endoplasmic reticulum or cell membrane into the cytosol.

The channel represents the increase in cytosolic $[Ca^{2+}]$ due to mobilisation by Ca^{2+} and IP_3. This term dominates the J_{pump} and J_{leak} terms during the peak of a Ca^{2+} wave:

$$J_{channel} = J_{max}[(\frac{[I]}{[I] + K_1})(1 - \frac{[C_s]}{C_{ser}})(\frac{[C]}{[C] + K_{act}})h]^3[1 - \frac{[C]}{C_{er}}], \tag{3.18}$$

J_{max} is the maximum channel current. $\frac{[I]}{[I]+K_1}(1 - \frac{[C_s]}{C_{ser}}$ represents IP_3 induced Ca^{2+} release having K_1 as the kinetic parameter, C_s as the Ca^{2+} concentration within the IP_3 sensitive pool and C_{ser} the initial size of the IP_3 sensitive Ca^{2+} pool. $[C]/([C] + K_{act})$ represents Ca^{2+} induced Ca^{2+} release with K_{act} as the kinetic parameter. $1 - \frac{[C]}{C_{er}}$ decreases the channel current when the

30

cytosolic concentration increases relative to that in the endoplasmic reticulum stores. h represents the inhibitory binding of Ca^{2+},

$$\frac{\partial h}{\partial t} = k_{on}[K_{inh} - ([C] + K_{inh})h],$$ (3.19)

and is initialised to its steady state

$$h_0 = \frac{K_{inh}}{[C]_0 + K_{inh}},$$ (3.20)

subsequently decreasing as cytosolic $[Ca^{2+}]$ increases and recovering as it decreases.

C_s represents the slow recovery IP_3 sensitive calcium store. Its initial value is zero and it depletes by increasing toward C_{ser}, the initial capacity of the IP_3 sensitive calcium store, according to:

$$\frac{\partial C_s}{\partial t} = J_{channel}(1 + \frac{[C]}{[C] + K_{act}} \frac{[I] + K_1}{[I] + \frac{C_s}{C_{ser}} - 1})^{-1}.$$ (3.21)

Active transport of Ca^{2+} into the endoplasmic reticulum from the cytosol is controlled by the calcium pumps:

$$J_{pump} = V_{max} \frac{[C]^2}{K_p^2 + [C]^2}.$$ (3.22)

The maximum rate for the pumps is determined by V_{max}. K_p is the dissociation constant and the Hill equation simulates two binding sites.

The Ca^{2+} leak refers to the release of calcium into the cytoplasm from the extracellular space or from intracellular stores as a result of normal metabolic activity:

$$J_{leak} = L(1 - \frac{[C]}{C_{er}}).$$ (3.23)

The leak is amplified when the concentration gradient between the intracellular stores and cytosol is greatest. The constant L determines the maximum leak.

The β term which scales the Ca^{2+} equation represents the effect of calcium buffering, in which calcium is bound to larger proteins rendering it inert.

$$\beta = (1 + \frac{[B]_{end}}{K_{end}} + \frac{[B]_{ex}K_{ex}}{([C] + K_{ex})^2})^{-1}.$$ (3.24)

The first term of 1 simply enables the effects of buffers to be ignored by setting the second and third terms to be zero. The second term refers to endogenous or static buffers, which do not diffuse, and the third term refers to exogenous or mobile buffers which do. In the present model the diffusion of buffered calcium is not considered.

3.2 Model Parameters

3.2.1 Parameter values

The parameters values listed in Table 3.1 are typical values used in calculations of the model. In most cases they have been taken from existing literature, both theoretical and experimental. Where the literature reports conflicting values for the parameters, or where parameter values are not precisely known, the reasons justifying the selection of each parameter are discussed below.

G-protein

Mahama and Linderman (1994) give the total number of G-protein molecules as 100,000 molecules per cell and the surface area of a cell as $2,200 \mu m^2$. From this the approximate G-protein concentration of 50 molecules per μm^2 has been calculated.

Bennett et al. (2005) use both the actual dissociation constant for ATP binding of Wu and Mori (1999) - which is around 10μM - and other factors influencing the effect of the P2Y receptors such as their density to comprise the effective dissociation constant K_{eff}. These other factors significantly affect the resulting K_{eff} value, giving a value between 25μM and 125μM. Here the actual dissociation constant is explicitly scaled by a further term to represent these effects so that $K_{eff} = K_R \sigma_R$.

IP_3

To determine the maximum possible rate of gap junctional intercellular diffusion the key factors are the extent of the coupling and the effectiveness of this coupling. The extent can be measured by four factors: the number of processes connecting two cells, the number of gap junctions per process, the number of channels per gap junction, and the fraction of channels that are open. There has been only limited study of these characteristics in glia. Rash et al. (2001) found that the number of gap junctions between two cells for each primary process (including the fibrous processes stemming from it) can be estimated at 4,000. The number of open channels per gap junction can be taken from Ransom and Ye (2005) as 200 although this value is somewhat imprecise. In using these in combination with the existing values for intercellular permeability (Höfer et al. 2002) a rate for the permeability per channel is determined.

ATP

Hubley et al. (1996) provide a range of values for the diffusion coefficient of ATP, dependent on environmental factors such as temperature. Between 25 and 40 degrees centigrade the range is $340\mu m^2 s^{-1}$ to $480\mu m^2 s^{-1}$. To maintain better consistency with previous models the lower value is used here.

The rate at which ectonucleotidases degrade ATP (and other adenonucleotides) in the extracellular space of glia has not been determined precisely. Dunwiddie et al. (1997) report a half life of $204 msec$ for the breakdown of ATP to adenosine (which includes the intermediate breakdowns to ADP and AMP). Dunwiddie's experiments were performed on the rat hippocampus and give a very high rate of degradation, greater than that apparently observed in Wang et al. (2000) and not consistent with Bennett et al. (2005). Lazarowski et al. (1997) provide a significantly slower half life of up to 25 minutes for ATP degradation in human astrocytes, comparable to the result of Ziganshin et al. (1996) for the *Xenopus laevis* oocyte which has an ATP half life of 33 minutes.

Since the results of Dunwiddie et al. (1997) do not fit the results of referenced experimental (Wang et al. 2000, Newman 2001) or theoretical studies (Bennett et al. 2005), the results of Lazarowski et al. (1997) were used. By fitting these results to the equation form in (3.15) the values for v_{deg} and A_{deg} have been derived.

Calcium

Miyawaki et al. (1997) provide a range of values for endoplasmic reticulum stored Ca^{2+} (C_{er}) of between 60 and 400. In line with Fink et al. (1999) the later value is used here.

Lytton et al. (1992) provide a set of values for the Ca^{2+} pumping rate (V_{max}) and dissociation constant (K_p). The values used by Fink et al. (1999), derived from the earlier paper, are used in this model.

Parameter	Symbol	Value	Source
G-protein			
G-protein ratio	K_G	$\frac{k_d}{k_a}$	
G-protein deactivation rate	k_d	$0.15 s^{-1}$	Lemon et al. (2003)
G-protein activation rate	k_a	$0.017 s^{-1}$	Lemon et al. (2003)
P2Y dissociation constant	K_R	$10\mu M$	Bennett et al. (2005)
P2Y density scaler	σ_R	1-2.5	Bennett et al. (2006)
Activation constant	δ_c	0	fit to experiment
IP$_3$			
IP$_3$ diffusion rate	D_{IP_3}	$280\mu m^2 s^{-1}$	Allbritton et al. (1992)
gap junctional			
G-protein concentration	G_{total}	$50\mu m^{-2}$	Mahama and Linderman (1994)
permeability for IP$_3$	P_{IP_3}	$1 - 5\mu m s^{-1}$	Höfer et al. (2002)
IP$_3$ production rate	ν_G	$4 \times 10^{-1}\mu M \mu m^2 s^{-1}$	Bennett et al. (2005)
IP$_3$ degradation rate	k_{deg}	$0.17 s^{-1}$	Atri et al. (1993)
Half saturation constant for			
calcium activation of PLCδ	K_{ca}	$0.3\mu M$	Höfer et al. (2002)
Maximal rate of PLCδ	ρ_{max}	$0.025\mu M s^{-1}$	Höfer et al. (2002)
Gap junctions per			
primary process	U_g	$4,000$	Rash et al. (2001)
Open channels per			
gap junction	U_o	200	Ransom and Ye (2005)
ATP			
ATP diffusion rate	D_{ATP}	$340\mu m^2 s^{-1}$	Hubley et al. (1996)
Ambient IP$_3$ concentration	I_{min}	$0.012 - 0.02\mu M$	Bennett et al. (2005)
ATP kinetic parameter	K_{rel}	$10\mu M$	Bennett et al. (2005)
ATP production rate	α_V	$2 \times 10^4\mu M s^{-1}$	Bennett et al. (2005)
ATP degradation rate	v_{deg}	$1\mu M s^{-1}$	Lazarowski et al. (1997)
ATP degradation parameter	A_{deg}	$5\mu M$	Lazarowski et al. (1997)
ATP release inhibitor	k_{loss}	$30 s^{-1}$	Bennett et al. (2005)
ATP release inhibitor recovery	χ_{repl}	$0 - 0.01 s^{-1}$	fit to experiment
Calcium			
Maximum channel current	J_{max}	$2,700\mu M s^{-1}$	Kupferman et al. (1997)
Saturation constant for IP3R	K_1	$0.03\mu M$	Fink et al. (1999)
Saturation constant for Ca^{2+}R	K_{act}	$0.17\mu M$	Fink et al. (1999)
Maximum free Ca^{2+} store			
in endoplasmic reticulum	C_{er}	$400\mu M$	Miyawaki et al. (1997)
Maximum free Ca^{2+} store			
in IP$_3$ sensitive pool	C_{ser}	$400\mu M$	fit to experiment
IP$_3$ channel kinetic parameter	k_{on}	$8\mu M^{-1}s^1$	Fink et al. (1999)
IP$_3$ background calcium	$[C]_0$	$0.05\mu M$	Fink et al. (1999)
IP$_3$ channel dissociation			
constant	K_{inh}	$0.1\mu M$	Fink et al. (1999)
Maximum pumping rate			
into ER	V_{max}	$5.85\mu M s^{-1}$	Lytton et al. (1992), Fink et al. (1999)
Pump dissociation constant	K_p	$0.24\mu M$	Lytton et al. (1992), Fink et al. (1999)
Leak constant	L	$0.0804\mu M s^{-1}$	Fink et al. (1999)
Endogenous (static) concentration			
to dissociation ratio	$\frac{B_{end}}{K_{end}}$	40	Xu et al. (1997)
Exogenous (mobile) buffer concentration	B_{ex}	$11.35\mu M$	Fink et al. (1999)

34

Chapter 4

Model Implementation

4.1 Numerical Technique

The present model simulates the reaction and diffusion of chemicals important to glial communication over a group of cells. In order to perform this simulation, the different biological structures (cellular somata, processes and the extracellular space) within the area must have their geometric and numerical characteristics discretised and quantified.

Constructing the geometry within the model consists of defining the location of each discretised portion of the structures within a 2 dimensional grid. The numerical methods are used to calculate the dynamic concentration changes of each of the chemicals at each of these grid positions. More detail on this is provided in the section below.

4.1.1 Geometry

The model is a collection of 2 dimensional shapes representing the extracellular space, cell somata and the protruding processes of cells. The basic structure is that representing the extracellular space (Fig. 4.1a) which is a rectangular grid subdivided into equally spaced squares. The primary purpose of the extracellular space is to provide a structure within which the concentration changes due to the reaction and diffusion of ATP can be calculated. Somata are represented within the model as hollow circles (Fig. 4.1b). Cells are discretised so that the perimeter of the cell is comprised of squares each of which corresponds to a square within the extracellular grid (Fig. 4.1c). Processes are represented as straight lines that protrude from the cell perimeter and connect with the extremity of another process (Fig. 4.1b). Gap junctions are defined at the connection of two processes, however due to their relatively small size they have no geometrical representation within the model.

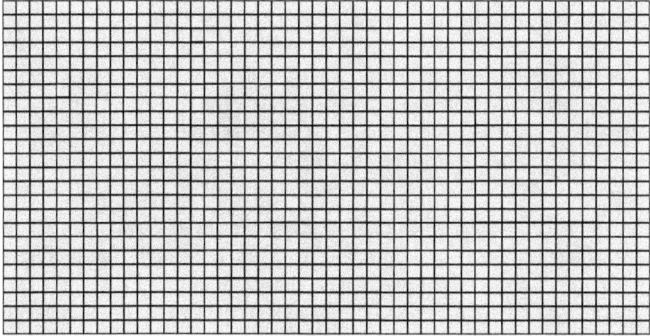

(a) Extracellular grid

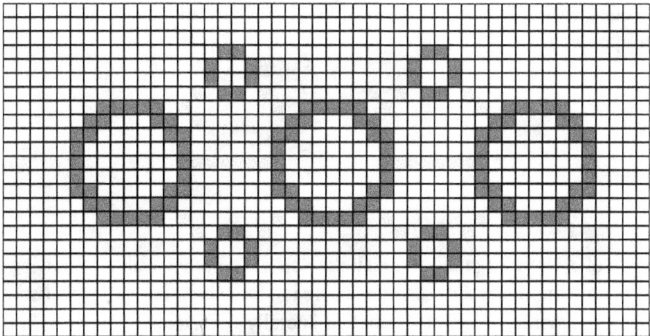

(b) Discretised cellular somata and processes

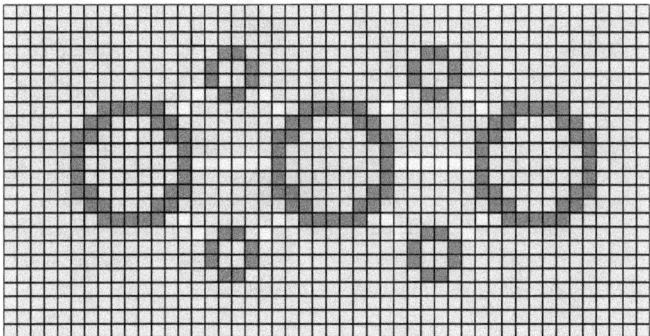

(c) Cellular somata and processes overlayed onto the extracellular grid

Figure 4.1: Geometry of simulation structures. Fig. 4.1a shows the discretisation of the 2 dimensional area of the simulation into equal sized square grids. In Fig. 4.1b the soma of each cell is discretised as a circle (blue squares). Processes (yellow squares) extend from the cell perimeters and connect to the process of another cell. Within Fig. 4.1c the grid squares used in Fig. 4.1b are each associated with a spatially corresponding grid square in Fig. 4.1a. Cells of different types may share gap junctional boundaries.

4.1.2   Numerical methods

The numerical methods used fall into two general categories: (1) calculating the effect of diffusion on ATP, IP_3 and Ca^{2+} concentrations within the geometric structures and (2) calculating the effect of chemical reactions both within and between the various structures.

As is common in numerical schemes of this type, the physical space represented by each simulation is divided into a series of grid squares (Fig. 4.1c). The simulations performed and described here using the present model use squares with an area of $1\mu m^2$. Each grid square records a single concentration value for each of the four chemicals considered in the model (ATP, IP_3, Ca^{2+} and G – protein). Reaction calculations consider the concentrations of multiple chemicals within a single spatial grid, whereas diffusion calculations reference the same chemical's concentration across surrounding grids. A description of how the calculations are made upon each of the described structures follows.

Extracellular space

The diffusion of ATP through the extracellular space structure is calculated using a 2 dimensional alternate direction implicit (ADI) scheme. There is a free-space boundary, realistic considering that a typical *in vivo* environment is not bounded laterally over areas of $\approx$ 1mm (a typical area used in the simulations). The diffusion calculations ignore the presence of cell structures, an aspect of the model intended to mimic the physiological capacity of ATP to diffuse around a cell in 3 dimensions and thus incorporate this in an appropriate way in the 2 dimensional geometry used by the simulations. In the model ATP is the only chemical to have a non-zero concentration within the extracellular space.

ATP is released into the environment from somata boundaries, which correspond to the cell wall. This is represented in the simulations by an ATP production calculation made at each grid square on the perimeter of the soma structures. Each of these grid squares in the cell correspond spatially to a grid square in the extracellular space grid (Sec. 4.1.1) and it is within the extracellular space that the resulting ATP concentration increase is applied. Once this increase is applied it will be included in the diffusion calculations at the next time step.

Due to the large number of grid squares within the extracellular space, and the use of the relatively expensive ADI algorithm (which is necessary to ensure the accuracy of the numerical calculation) the time taken to solve the diffusion effects within the extracellular grid generally accounts for the majority of the simulations' execution time within simulations containing less than 30 cells.

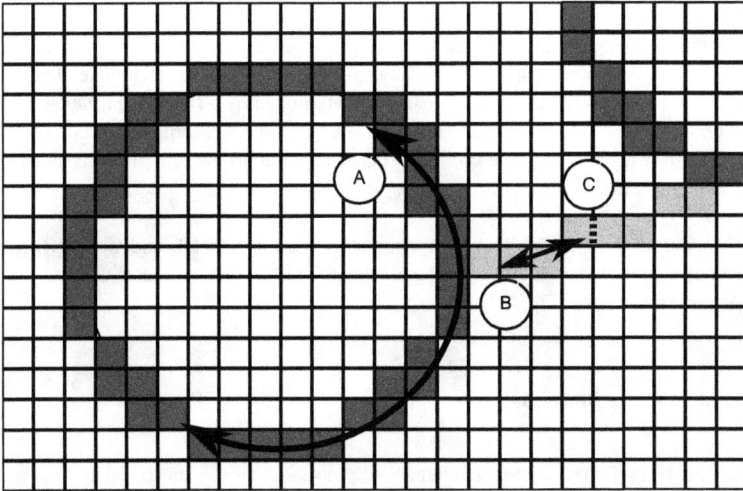

Figure 4.2: Overview of numerics for cellular structures. Diffusion is around the cell wall (A) and through a line with boundary conditions for each process (B - C). A function at the process boundary with the cell (B) determines the IP_3 concentration using standard diffusion calculations whereas the concentrations on either side of the gap junction boundary (C) between the two processes are determined by the attributes of the gap junctions and processes such as permeability to IP_3 and the number of open gap junctions.

Cellular somata

Each soma is treated independently within the calculations. For the purposes of the numeric solution a soma consists of a perimeter only, as production calculations are predominantly made at the perimeter. Originally calculations were performed over the entire cell, including the internal space, however it was found that the difference in the results was marginal and the increase in execution time was significant. Due to this the more simplified numerical representation of cells has been used.

Somata may contain non-zero concentrations of IP_3, Ca^{2+} and $G - protein$. At each time step reaction equations are calculated for each grid square to determine the production and possible degradation of each of these chemicals using the forward Euler technique. For example, the change in $[IP_3]$ at each grid square is partially determined by a function of the current G-protein concentration (Eq. 3.7) within the same grid square only. ATP production is also calculated at the cell wall grid (it is dependent on the IP_3 concentration) and this quantity is added into the corresponding extracellular grid squares.

Diffusion is calculated within each soma structure for both IP_3 and Ca^{2+}. Diffusion is calculated separately for each of these chemicals around the cell perimeter using a 1 dimensional Dufort-Frankel scheme (Fig. 4.2).

Processes and gap junctions

The equations used to simulate the influence of processes and somata are calculated independently within this model. A process is modelled as a line of grid squares that connect on one end to a grid square on the cell perimeter and at the other end to another process (Fig. 4.2). Within the line of grid squares representing the process, the diffusion of IP_3 is calculated using a 1 dimensional Dufort-Frankel scheme with boundary values determined using functions dependent upon the $[IP_3]$ in the corresponding cell perimeter grid or the connecting process grid square (Fig. 4.2). The function at the soma-side boundary acts simply to connect the two IP_3 diffusion calculations (i.e. the one for the soma and the other for the process) while the function at the boundary where the processes connect accounts for the effect of gap junctions (see Eq. 3.12) as well as diffusion.

4.2 Technical Environment

The model has been developed using the Java programming language (Gosling 2000) due to its good balance of execution speed and development time when compared with Matlab, Fortran and C. It has been tested on Microsoft Windows and a variety of Unix platforms.

The SSJ package (L'Ecuyer et al. 2002) is used to generate stochastic variation in gap junctional permeability and the kxml package (Haustein 2005) used to load the program parameters.

Chapter 5

Comparison of Intercellular and Extracellular Effects in Glial Clusters

A principal motivation in the development of the present model is to facilitate comparison of the effects of intercellular and extracellular pathways within a glial cluster. A series of three simulations have been constructed in which (1) both pathways are active, (2) only the extracellular pathway is active and (3) only the intercellular pathway is active. The resulting time-courses are then compared to elucidate the relative contribution of each pathway.

The comparisons are made using a dense and strongly connected cluster of cells. It should be noted that the structure, the cellular morphology and the particular parameter values used will result in different degrees of influence from each of the pathways. For example, it is obvious that in a cluster of cells with minimal gap junctional coupling the extracellular pathway will always dominate, or in a cluster where the ATP degradation is very high then the intercellular pathway will always dominate. These simulations are used to determine how using both pathways differs from using only one; for example to determine whether concentrations in a combined simulation are greater than, equal to or less than the sum of the concentrations in the individual simulations.

5.1   Configuration

The cluster of cells is configured as a square matrix of eighty-one glial cells each of radius $10\mu m$. In each simulation the central cell is initialised for two seconds. Gap junctions are established between vertical, horizontal and diagonal neighbours and the cells are spaced $40\mu m$ apart (from cell centre to cell centre) resulting in $20\mu m$ of extracellular space separating neighbouring cell boundaries at their closest proximity.

5.2 Parameters

Parameters are within the range defined in Table 3.1, with values selected that produce relatively small waves in order to study the effects more closely. In order to simulate the deactivation of the extracellular pathway the rate of active activation of G-protein is set to zero, and when the intercellular pathway is deactivated this is simulated by setting the permeability at connexons to zero.

Initialisation is established within the extracellular-only simulation by a 2 second pulse of ATP at $80\mu Ms^{-1}$ and within the intercellular-only simulation by a 2 second pulse of IP_3 at $0.5\mu Ms^{-1}$. The simulation with both mechanisms includes both of these initialisation terms.

5.3 Results

To compare the results of the simulations the concentration of IP_3 has been plotted. IP_3 has been chosen as it is the easiest to compare amongst all three simulations since ATP is not relevant when extracellular diffusion is not used and Ca^{2+} concentration is dependent on IP_3. As expected, the results indicate that when both pathways are active the overall concentration and radius of the IP_3 wave is increased (Fig. 5.1). It is relevant to observe from Fig. 5.1 how column (A), which displays the results of the simulation containing both intercellular and extracellular mechanisms, relates to columns (B) and (C), which display the results of the extracellular only and intercellular only simulations respectively. At 2 seconds, when the initial release is terminated, it is apparent that the effects of intercellular communication are dominating the combined IP_3 concentrations. At this time the radius and concentration of the non-initialised cells are equivalent between (A) and (C). Conversely, the concentration in (B) is higher for the initialised cell and lower for non-initialised cells than in (A). At 4 seconds the impact of extracellular diffusion is more apparent in (A) with those cells exhibiting elevated concentrations in (B) also having elevated concentrations in (A). By 8 seconds concentrations in (A) have exceeded those in (C) within all cells although the radius is similar between the two simulations. Interestingly the concentration in the central cells of (B) is still higher than that in the corresponding cells of (A); however the wave radius is much smaller in (B). By 16 seconds the concentration is decreasing in all 3 simulations at different rates; the two simulations with extracellular diffusion pathways are maintaining somewhat elevated concentrations with (A) still having a much greater radius than (B). By contrast (C) is nearly completely returned to the pre-existing equilibrium concentration.

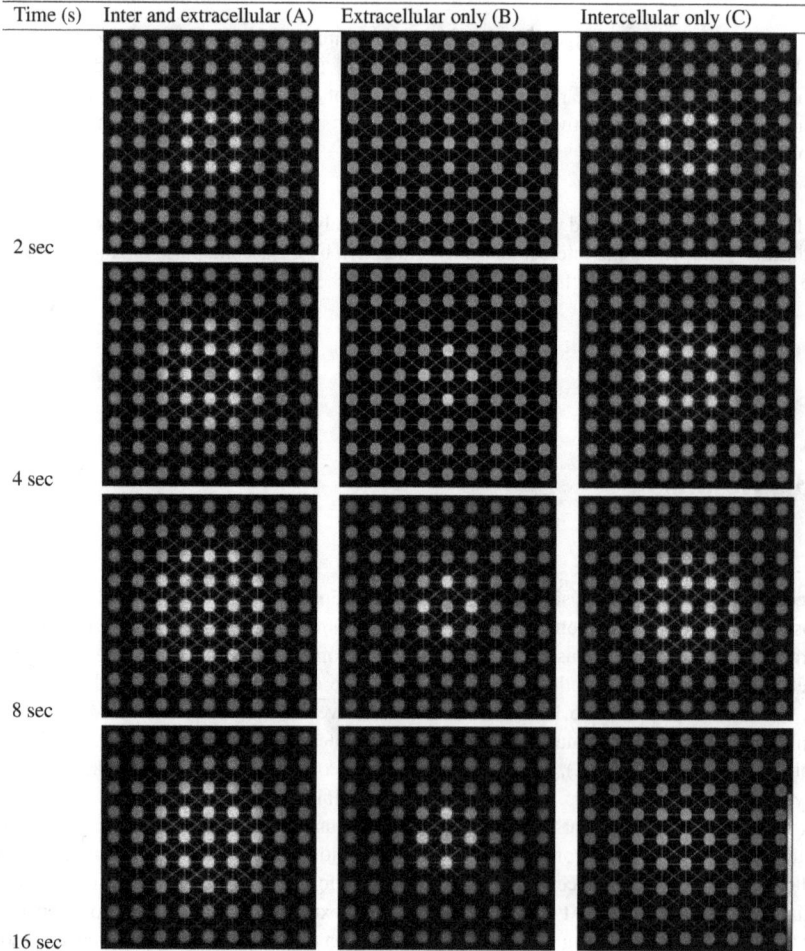

Figure 5.1: IP$_3$ concentration at selected times courses for simulations using (A) both intercellular and extracellular communication, (B) only extracellular communication and (C) only intercellular communication. Scale bar in bottom right cell has a maximum at 0.05μM.

IP3 concentration in central cell

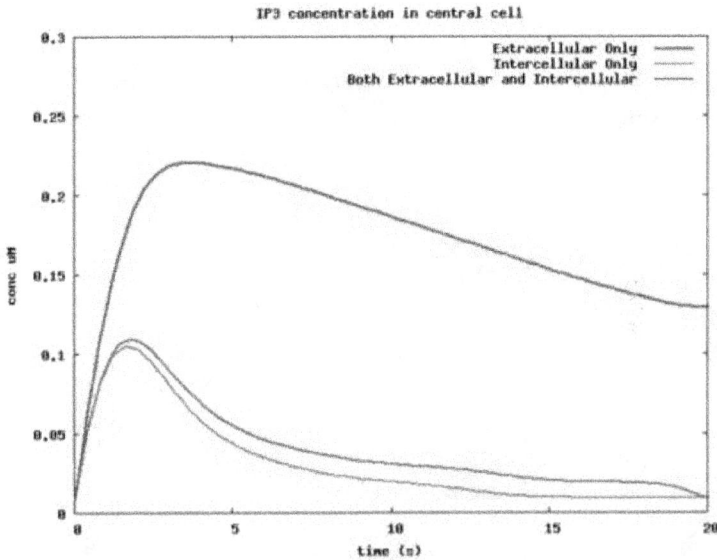

Figure 5.2: IP$_3$ concentrations over time for the initialised cell in the three different simulations. The peak concentration in the extracellular only simulation exceeds that in the simulation with both pathways, a result that is due to the faster dispersal of initialised IP$_3$ via the permeable gap junctions.

IP3 concentration in neighbour to central cell

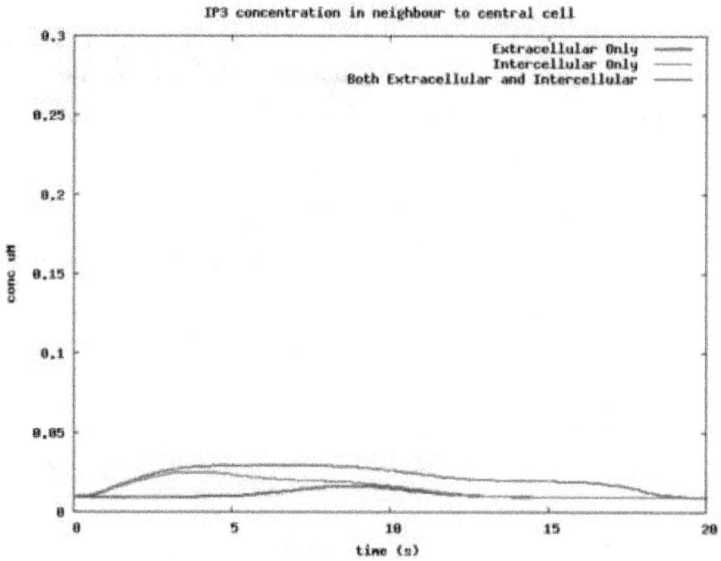

Figure 5.3: IP$_3$ concentrations over time for an immediate neighbour to the initialised cell in the three different simulations. The combined simulation produces the greatest peak concentration in this cell, unlike in the initialised cell in which the extracellular only simulation produces the greatest concentration.

5.4 Discussion

Fig. 5.1 suggests that extracellular communication has a tendency to increase the concentration and the duration of IP_3 whereas intercellular communication tends to increase the radius. It should be noted however that drawing general conclusions from these particular results is problematic since with different parameters the results may be quite different - for example with a significantly higher rate of ATP production (or lower ATP degradation rate) the extracellular only results would have a far greater radius.

The results displayed in Fig. 5.1 suggest that when both extracellular and intercellular pathways are used in a simulation the effect is qualitatively similar to adding the contributions from both the simulations in which only one of the pathways is used. Due to this the radius is greater, the duration is longer, and most cells' concentration is greater in the combined simulation. This is expected as the total production of chemical is being increased by including both pathways.

Fig. 5.2 demonstrates that the cumulative effect of including both pathways is, while generally additive, not completely so. The peak IP_3 is greater in the extracellular only plot than it is in the combined plot, in fact the peak IP_3 concentration in the combined plot is very similar to that in the intercellular only plot. The explanation for the lower peak IP_3 concentration in the combined simulation compared to the extracellular only simulation is that the diffusion of IP_3 into surrounding cells due to the permeable gap junctions decreases the total IP_3 in the initiating cell. Fig. 5.3, which plots the IP_3 concentrations in one of the cells immediately neighbouring the centre cell against time for each of the simulations, shows that using both extracellular and intercellular pathways will increase the total concentration in cells in which external application (i.e. initialisation) is not applied.

Chapter 6

Comparison with Existing Models

In order to evaluate the accuracy of the present model, calculations from three previously published glia models (Sneyd et al. 1995, Höfer et al. 2002, Bennett et al. 2005) were replicated. These three models were selected because they each focus on a distinct mechanism of Ca^{2+} wave propagation. The first uses passive, gap junctional diffusion of non-regenerative IP_3 to release Ca^{2+} (Sneyd et al. 1995), the second adds a regenerative component to the wave by including Ca^{2+} induced IP_3 release (Höfer et al. 2002) and the last model describes diffusion of ATP through the extracellular space resulting in both the release of Ca^{2+} from intracellular stores and the subsequent extracellular release of ATP from cells (Bennett et al. 2005). Combined, these three models simulate the principal mechanisms of Ca^{2+} wave propagation within glial cell networks. The following chapter demonstrates the present model's capacity to produce results similar to each of these existing models and thereby its potential to accurately simulate Ca^{2+} waves in networks of glial cells exhibiting *all* of these mechanisms. Results will not be identically replicated as the underlying equations and structure of the present model differs from the previous models, nevertheless, similar results have been obtained to all three previous models.

6.1 Comparison with Sneyd Wetton Charles Sanderson (1995)

As discussed in Sec. 2.10, Sneyd et al. (1995) present a model in which IP_3 diffuses from a central cell through gap junctions into a two dimensional network of airway epithelial cells. The elevated $[IP_3]$ induces the release of Ca^{2+} and is not regenerated. This provides a constraint on the distance that the Ca^{2+} wave may travel.

47

6.1.1 Configuration

To the extent possible, the parameters from Sneyd et al. (1995) were used in the present model. The initial step was to define a grid with sides of length 240μm containing sixty four cells laid out in a square pattern (Fig. 6.1) in which gap junctions were added horizontally and vertically such that internal cells share gap junctions with four neighbours each.

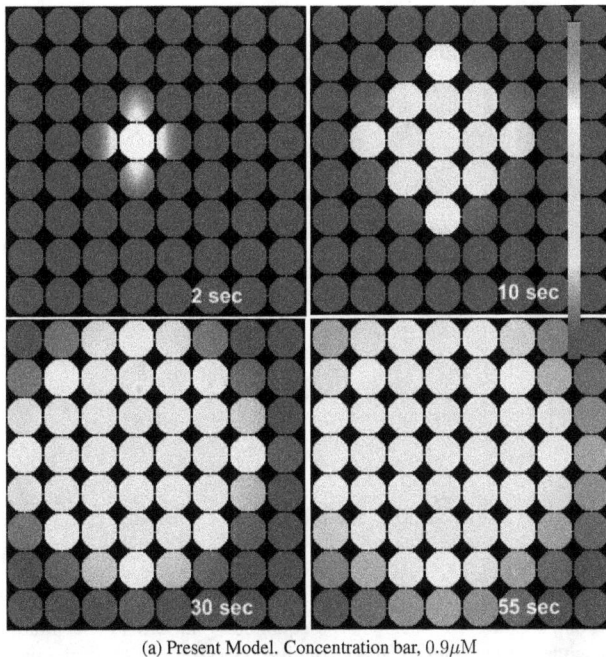

(a) Present Model. Concentration bar, 0.9μM

Figure 6.1: Cellular grid at four different times. $[Ca^{2+}]$ is displayed within individual cells (note that cells are circular in the present model rather than the more usual square representation). The calcium wave is initiated by applying 0.72μMs^{-1} of IP$_3$ for 15 seconds to the central cell.

Since ATP is absent from the model, the parameter ν_G in Eq. 3.7 is set to zero. This prevents IP$_3$ from being released due to the action of ATP and thereby disables activity in the PLCβ pathway. Likewise, the PLCδ pathway's production of IP$_3$ is disabled by setting the ρ_{max} parameter in Eq. 3.8 to zero. With these two pathways turned off, the only mechanism able to produce an increase in the IP$_3$ concentration is the initial release in the central cell. In this calculation, $0.72\mu Ms^{-1}$ of IP$_3$ was added to cell 1 (see Fig. 6.1) for 15 seconds.

The sets of equations used in the present model are not identical to those given by Sneyd et al. (1995). The degradation term for IP$_3$ of Sneyd et al. (1995) saturates and thus differs from the linear term in Eq. 3.9. By plotting the concentration time-courses of both terms, given an appropriate initial concentration (Fig. 6.2) and the actual degradation rate over a range of concentrations (Fig. 6.3), the value of $0.025\mu\text{ms}^{-1}$ was determined to be most appropriate for the parameter k_{deg} in Eq. 3.9. The effect of using a linear degradation as opposed to a saturation equation will be that higher concentrations degrade relatively rapidly and lower concentrations relatively slowly. The impact of this difference is discussed later in this section.

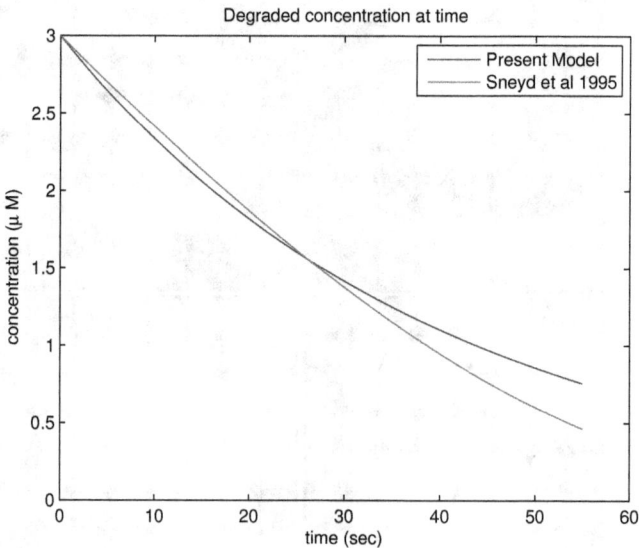

Figure 6.2: Comparison of IP_3 degradation equations - an initial concentration is decayed over time. The degradation constant for the saturation type degradation in the model of Sneyd et al. (1995) is $0.08\mu\text{M}$ and the linear degradation rate in the present model is 0.025s^{-1}. It is apparent that linear degradation is greater at high concentrations and smaller at lower concentrations.

The equations describing the Ca^{2+} dynamics are also somewhat different between the two models. Sneyd et al. (1995) do not include an explicit buffer term in their Eq. 2 and so the β term in Eq. 3.24, which defines the effect of endogenous and exogenous buffers, is set to a value of 1 which eliminates any effect from the buffers. The J_{leak} term (Eq. 3.23) is essentially the same between the two models when $C_{er} \gg [C]$ and L is equated to the β of Sneyd et al. (1995), so L is set to $0.15\mu\text{Ms}^{-1}$. The J_{pump} term (Eq. 3.22) is exactly the same in the two models. The $J_{channel}$ (or J_{flux}) term (Eq. 3.18) differs, particularly in the treatment of the inactivation of IP_3 receptors and the rates for maximal channel current. Since it is not possible to simply equate parameters in this case the parameters are kept as defined in section Sec. 3.2.

The intercellular permeability (P_{ip3}) for the gap junctions is set to $2\mu\text{ms}^{-1}$ in order to conform

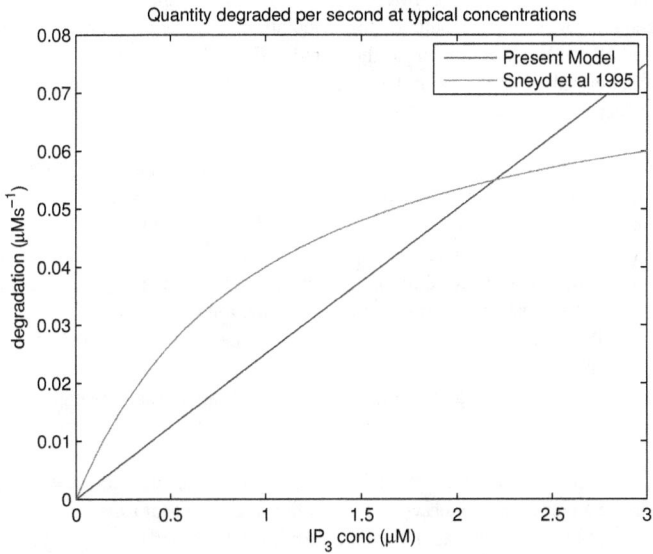

Figure 6.3: Comparison of IP$_3$ degradation equations - plots of the actual decay rates at typical concentrations

to the value of Sneyd et al. (1995).

6.1.2 Results

The time-courses for [IP$_3$] are given in Fig. 6.4 and show good agreement between the two models. The principal factors in determining the concentration of IP$_3$ in the model of Sneyd et al. (1995) are: the initial release of IP$_3$, the diffusion rate of IP$_3$, the permeability of gap junctions and the IP$_3$ degradation rate. Each of the first three factors take identical values in each model so this result is to be expected if the minor differences in structure and morphology of the cell networks are of little significance to the results of the calculations. These differences include the square cells of Sneyd et al. (1995) compared to the round cells in the present model. The difference in the degradation calculations has been discussed and as noted this difference has been minimised by prudent selection of parameter values.

The [Ca^{2+}] time-courses in Fig. 6.5 exhibit differences in the models. The concentrations in the present model peak at lower concentrations than those of Sneyd et al. (1995) and there is a spike evident in the initial peak for the present model's central cell that is absent in the plot from Sneyd et al. (1995). The differences in the [Ca^{2+}] time-courses can be explained by reference to the differences in the equations used in the models. The present model (see Eq. 3.17) is based on Fink et al. (1999), who use a much higher rate of production of Ca^{2+} from the $J_{channel}$ term (Eq. 3.18) and an inhibition term (Eq. 3.19) that slows Ca^{2+} production commensurately faster. This explains the initial spike in the first cell, as observed in the present model (Fig. 6.5). The [Ca^{2+}] time-courses indicate that the wave radius and velocity are approximately equal between the two models.

The Ca^{2+} concentration across all cells in the grids at four distinct times are compared in Fig. 6.1. The concentrations match well, though the final panel (at time 55 seconds) shows that peripheral cells maintain an elevated concentration in the present model for longer than Sneyd et al. (1995), though the concentrations are decreasing. As explained above, this is due to the different forms for the IP$_3$ degradation terms that result in relatively slower degradation at low concentrations for the current model. The wave radii produced by each of the models are the same up to thirty seconds, which is the period during which the wave is expanding. Differences between the models emerge after this time, as can be seen in the 55 second panels, once degradation starts to dominate the concentration changes.

6.1.3 Discussion

The results of Sneyd et al. (1995) and the present model, for a similar set of parameters over a similarly structured network of cells, have been compared. The two models lead to essentially identical results for [IP$_3$] and closely matching results for [Ca^{2+}]. Where the [Ca^{2+}] results differ

51

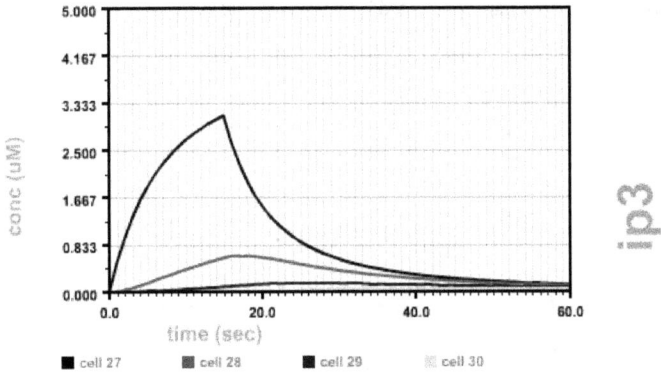

(a) Present Model

Figure 6.4: [IP$_3$] time-courses

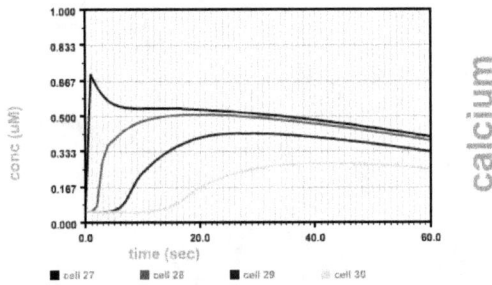

(a) Present Model

Figure 6.5: [Ca^{2+}] time-courses.

it is due to the use of more recent equations (especially those of Fink et al. (1999)) to model the dynamics and the effect of the different degradation terms at low IP_3 concentrations. Despite these differences, the similarities between models in regards to the radius and velocity of the waves and the time-course of both $[Ca^{2+}]$ and $[IP_3]$ all indicate that the present model successfully replicates the passive diffusion scenario presented by Sneyd et al. (1995).

6.2 Comparison with Höfer Venance Giaume (2002)

Höfer et al. (2002) modelled a network of cells in which IP_3 and Ca^{2+} interactions produce a regenerative Ca^{2+} wave (Sec. 2.11). The most significant difference from the passive diffusion model of Sneyd et al. (1995) is that $[IP_3]$, in addition to being depleted over time by diffusion and degradation, is regenerated by transient increases in Ca^{2+} concentration. The most significant impact of this difference is that the model has the potential to produce Ca^{2+} waves of much greater radius; indeed for some parameter values the wave radius is infinite.

Two of the principal results from Höfer et al. (2002) are the effect of heterogeneous gap junction coupling strengths on the formation of preferential pathways for Ca^{2+} waves and the combined impact of the PLCδ rate and the IP_3 permeability through gap junctions on the type of Ca^{2+} signals produced. This section will demonstrate that the present model exhibits the same capacity for forming preferential pathways for Ca^{2+} waves and that the formation of either regenerative, limited regenerative or diffusion-like Ca^{2+} waves is dependent on the parameter selection for PLCδ and for IP_3 permeability.

6.2.1 Configuration

A square eighty one cell network of astrocytes was constructed in which each astrocyte is connected via gap junctions to its horizontal and vertical neighbours (Fig. 6.6). Non-overlapping processes extend from the somata of these neighbouring cells and form gap junctions at their extremities. This is different to the contiguous square layout of the astrocytes defined by Höfer et al. (2002) but better conforms to the morphology of astrocytes.

Parameters have been either taken directly from Table 1 in Höfer et al. (2002) or fitted to the results that they reported.

6.2.2 Results

Preferential pathways

Höfer et al. (2002) identified that variations in the strength of gap junctional coupling produce irregular (i.e. non-concentric) intercellular calcium waves. The different permeabilities at each gap junction are not explicitly given by Höfer et al. (2002) but are derived statistically from existing data on gap junctional conductance. As conductance and permeability are linearly related (Verselis et al. 1986), variations in conductance throughout the cell network were simulated by randomly assigning different gap junctional permeabilities. The random permeabilities were determined

Permeability ($\mu M s^{-1}$)	Weight
0.0	0.4
1.5	0.2
3.0	0.15
4.5	0.05
6.0	0.2

Table 6.1: Details for discrete distribution used in forming preferential pathways. The weights for the permeabilities are taken from Höfer et al. (2002) Fig. 7a. The permeabilities are estimated from the range established in the present model (Fig. 6.7).

from a discrete distribution skewed toward low values (see Table 6.1 for details of the distribution). Using this technique, preferential pathways were formed in the present model; a typical set of results is presented in Fig. 6.6.

The present model was run multiple times for the same distribution and each set of calculations produced were quantitatively different. Three distinct types of results became apparent: one in which the [Ca^{2+}] throughout the entire network of cells becomes (asymmetrically) elevated; another in which the Ca^{2+} wave spread throughout a sub-section of the network but avoids other sub-sections closer to the initialised cell; and one in which the Ca^{2+} wave was confined to a small area around the initially stimulated cell.

Signal type

Höfer et al. (2002) identified the rate of PLCδ activity (ρ_{max} in Eq. 3.8) and the permeability of the gap junctions to IP$_3$ (P_{ip3} in Eq. 3.14) of gap junctions as critical parameters in determining whether the type of signal produced by an initialising stimulus is finitely regenerative, infinitely regenerative or diffusion-like. A series of calculations were performed using the present model in which ρ_{max} was adjusted as was P_{ip3}. It was found that the form of Fig. 4 from Höfer et al. (2002) was qualitatively reproduced in the present model (Fig. 6.7).

The calculations indicated that qualitative changes in the signal type occur along boundaries in which one parameter increases as the other decreases. Furthermore, the range of values for which limited regenerative waves (waves which extended beyond the radius of diffusive waves but which were nevertheless finite) occur grows as permeability is increased.

6.2.3 Discussion

By using a comparable distribution of gap junction coupling strengths the present model has produced qualitatively similar preferential pathways to those of Höfer et al. (2002). These authors

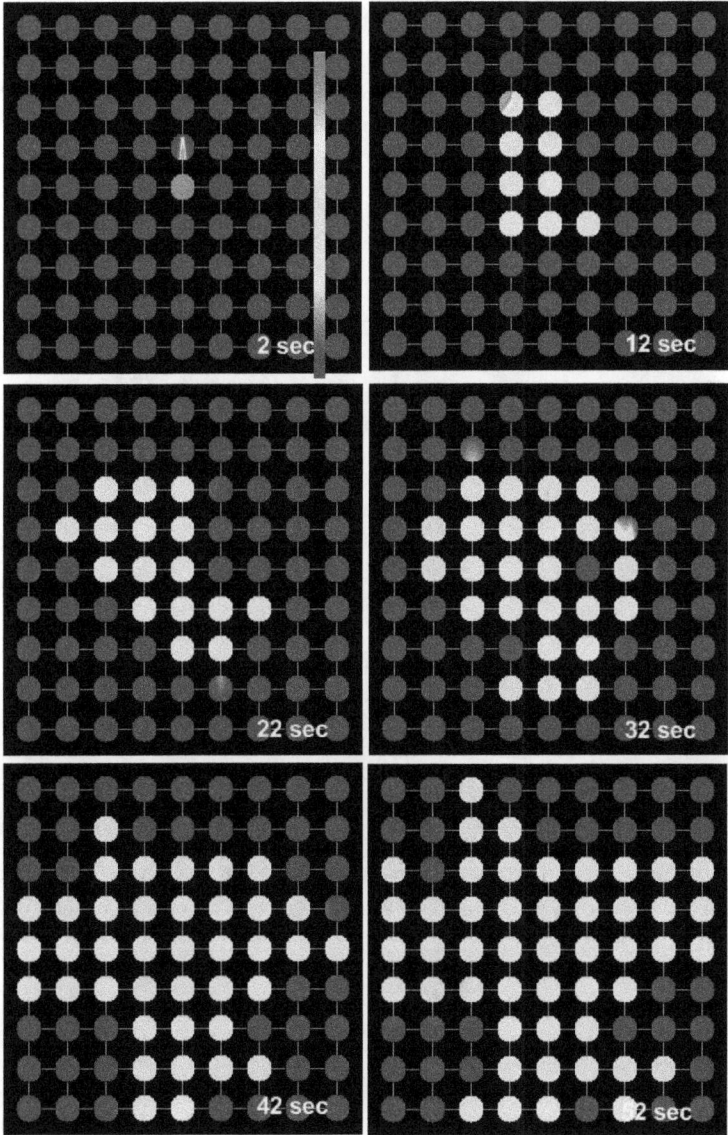

Figure 6.6: Heterogeneous gap junction coupling strengths produce preferential pathways for calcium waves. Coupling strengths were randomly assigned to each gap junction according to the distribution defined in Table 6.1. Concentration bar, $1\mu M$.

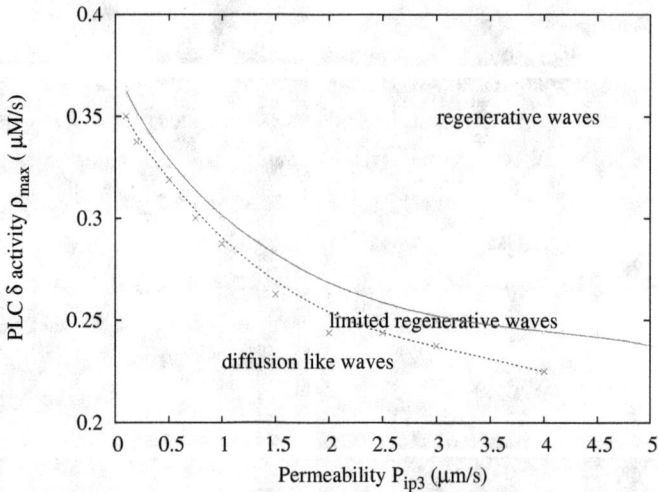

(a) Present Model. Stars and crosses indicate sample points of calculations, lines have been fitted to these points.

Figure 6.7: Signal type dependence on PLCδ activity and IP$_3$ permeability. The labels indicate regions in which the parameters produce waves of that type. It follows the form of Fig.4 from Höfer et al. (2002) though the PLCδ activity rate varies (see discussion).

reported that they were unable to form these preferential pathways when varying other parameters randomly as the waves formed were essentially concentric, an effect also found when randomly varying other parameters in the present model. The present model also formed near concentric waves when the probability distribution of permeabilities was symmetric. One interpretation of these results is that preferential pathways are more likely to form when there are greater differences in the total permeabilities of small groups of cells within a cluster. When this condition is not met and regions of neighbouring cells tend to have similar total permeabilities, then the wave velocity in different regions tends to average out and distinct pathways are not formed.

It should be noted that the form of Eq. 3.14 in the present model is such that, in terms of its effect on the flux between two cells, varying the permeability of a gap junction channel is equivalent to varying the number of open channels. Due to this, results from the present model reflect the effect of differences in the total coupling strength of gap junctions rather than the effect of differences in the permeability of individual gap junctions. Furthermore whereas Höfer et al. (2002) define contiguous boundaries between cells, meaning that every point along the cell wall is engaged in intercellular diffusion, the present model restricts this to gap junctions at connected processes as this conforms better to the biology of glia.

The same form as in the plot of signal types displayed as Fig. 4 of Höfer et al. (2002) is clearly produced by this model. The difference in the PLCδ activity rates examined may be due to a number of factors: there are different morphologies between the models; there are disparate forms for the calcium equations; and there are differences in what the intercellular flux for a particular permeability rate, as described in the previous paragraph, is between the two models. The significant result is that signal type is determined by the intracellular production rate of IP$_3$ and the speed with which it travels intercellularly.

These two results from Höfer et al. (2002) were chosen to be replicated in the present model in order to demonstrate its capacity to produce results other than concentration time-courses and its ability to do so in a way that conforms with the results of a gap junction oriented model such as that of Höfer et al. (2002).

6.3 Comparison with Bennett Farnell Gibson (2005)

Bennett et al. (2005) present a glial model in which a regenerative Ca^{2+} wave is mediated by extracellular diffusion of ATP (Sec. 2.13). This differs considerably from the previously replicated models which described intercellular communication only. The other principal difference of this model, both to existing models and the present model, is that it calculates over three dimensions rather than the more usual two dimensions.

6.3.1 Configuration

The parameters used to produce Fig. 4 Col.A in Bennett et al. (2005) were applied to the current model where possible. A $1,010\mu$m by 60μm rectangular grid containing 19 identical cells arranged in a single lane containing cells with a radius of 12.5μm and having centres 50μm apart was defined (Fig. 6.8). The centre cell is initialised with 80μMs^{-1} of ATP for one second. The K_R and σ_R values of Eq. 3.15 are set to 10 and 2.5 respectively, to match the K_R value of 25μM defined by Bennett et al. (2005) in their Fig. 2. IP$_3$ diffusion occurs at a rate of 280μm^{2}s^{-1} and the degradation rate for IP$_3$ (k_{deg}) is increased to 1.25s^{-1}. G_{total} and ν_G (Eq. 3.9) are set to match the r_h^* value ($2 \times 10^{-14}\mu mol\mu m^{-2}s^{-1}$) of Bennett et al. (2005). Calcium parameters are identical to Bennett et al. (2005).

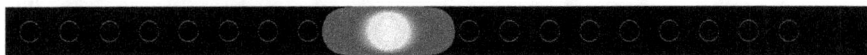

Figure 6.8: Structure of model for replication of Bennett et al. (2005). Astrocytes are represented as circles within the image.

Two changes to parameter values were introduced in order to fit the previous results more accurately. Values for the extracellular degradation of ATP were included ($v_{deg} = 1$ and $A_{deg} = 5$), increasing the rate of extracellular depletion for ATP and the parameter α_V, which determines the production rate of ATP, was increased to $40,000$ from $4,000$. These changes act both to increase the rate of production of ATP and conversely to increase its rate of depletion. The effect is to elevate the concentration of ATP at the cell wall, thereby encouraging the activation of G-protein by the bound purinergic receptors, while maintaining a similar ATP concentration throughout the extracellular space. It is likely that this is required due to the 2 dimensional nature of this model compared to the 3 dimensional nature of the model of Bennett et al. (2005) which gives a larger surface area for the cell.

As in the calculations of Bennett et al. (2005), no gap junctions are included in the model.

6.3.2 Results

The results from the ATP calculations of both models are compared in Fig. 6.9. They demonstrate that the range, peak concentrations and velocity of the ATP wave are similar in both models. The arrival time is principally determined by the speed of diffusion however the peaks are dependent on the subsequent IP_3 mediated release of ATP. The associated curves for ATP store depletion (Fig. 6.10) are also very similar with respect to both the slope and to the concentrations.

The plots of IP_3 (Fig. 6.11) bear a close resemblance in their time-courses. The result that both ATP and IP_3 concentrations are similar over the time range is significant, as these two chemicals are the primary agents of both regeneration and propagation within the model of Bennett et al. (2005). As the Eq. 1 in Fink et al. (1999) is closely followed in both Bennett et al. (2005) and the present model, it is to be expected that the Ca^{2+} plots (Fig. 6.12) are in close agreement given the strong match of the IP_3 and ATP time-courses in the respective models. Any differences are likely to be attributable principally to the differences in the IP_3 concentrations rather than to variations in the Ca^{2+} equations.

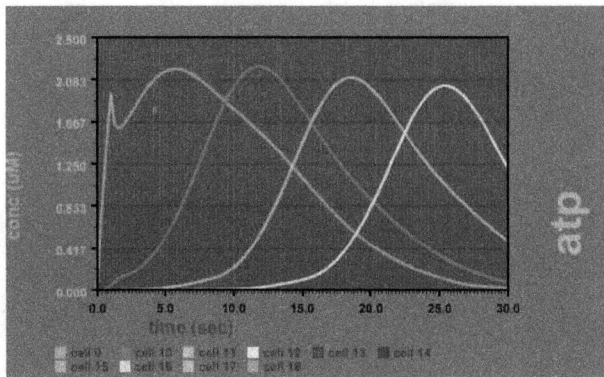

(a) Present Model

Figure 6.9: [ATP] time-courses for 4 cells. The concentrations of the cells and velocities of the waves are in good agreement, however the slight increase in the peak concentration of downstream cells of Bennett et al. (2005) is not apparent in the present model.

6.3.3 Discussion

The most significant difference between the models is that of dimension - the present model is only two dimensional while Bennett et al. (2005) present a three dimensional model. Nevertheless, their calculations are of three dimensional cells acting in a two dimensional layer (that is all cells are

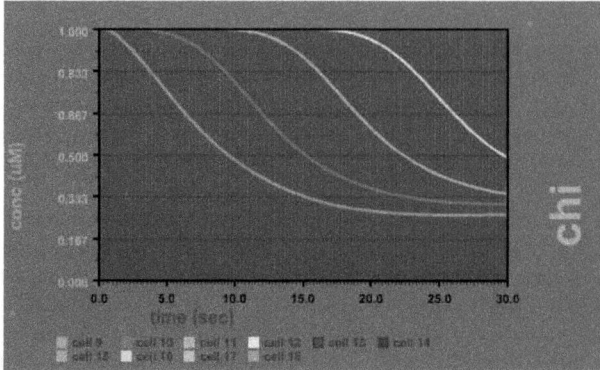

(a) Present Model

Figure 6.10: ATP store depletion ($\chi(t)$) time-courses for 4 cells. The time-courses have similar minimum values, however the rate of depletion is greater in the present model than to Bennett et al. (2005).

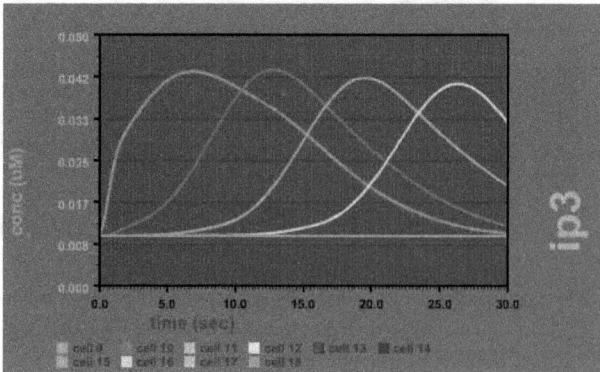

(a) Present Model

Figure 6.11: [IP$_3$] time-courses for 4 cells between models. The velocities and shapes of time-courses of the models are similar, however the peak concentration is greater in the present model as compared with Bennett et al. (2005). This is possibly due to the 2 dimensional nature of the present model, which measures IP$_3$ concentration at the cell wall, not allowing IP$_3$ to diffuse into the internal cytoplasm as rapidly as the 3 dimensional model of Bennett et al. (2005).

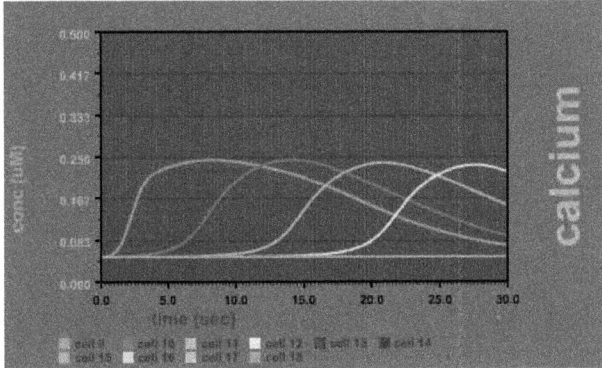

(a) This Model

Figure 6.12: $[Ca^{2+}]$ time-courses for 4 cells. There is good agreement in the peak concentrations and velocities of the two waves. The present model produces a less rapid initial increase in concentration than Bennett et al. (2005) however. This may be due to differences in the respective IP_3 time-courses.

at the same height) and so the structure of the cell network in both models is broadly equivalent. The other principal difference in the models is that the present model uses circular cells whereas Bennett et al. (2005) use cubes to represent cells.

The ability of the present model to successfully replicate the results of Bennett et al. (2005), despite the differences explained previously, is enhanced by the similarity of the equations used in the calculations. It is significant that calculations using a 2 dimensional model can closely match those using a 3 dimensional model, since the computation time can be significantly decreased by reducing the number of dimensions.

6.4 Summary of Comparison to Existing Models

While the results were not precisely equal, in each of the three papers compared the present model was successful in replicating the important features. This demonstrates that the model is able to provide the same insights as existing models into glial cell communication. The novel aspect of the present model, the capacity to combine these attributes together in order to simulate a wider range of glial cell activity, is explored in the following section.

Chapter 7

Simulation of Experimental Observations

There are no existing theoretical models of chemical communication within glial cell clusters that incorporate both a regenerative extracellular pathway and a regenerative intercellular pathway. The most complete existing model is the stochastic model presented within Iacobas et al. (2006) which includes both an intercellular and an extracellular pathway; however the extracellular ATP is not regenerative (see Sec. 2.14). To evaluate the ability of the present model to simulate the combined effect of these pathways it is necessary to compare simulation results to experimental data.

7.1 Comparison with Newman (2001)

As reviewed in section Sec. 2.6, Newman (2001) details observations of Ca^{2+} and ATP waves in a network of retinal glial cells in which both extracellular diffusion and intercellular gap junctions are involved in producing a Ca^{2+} wave. Existing models cannot adequately model this situation due to the combination of different interactions that occur. These experimental results are ideal for evaluation of the present model as they evaluate the relative influence of each pathway by conditioning the glial cluster with antagonists and enzymes that selectively block the effects of the pathways. Additionally, as the experimental results make clear the importance of both astrocytes and Müller cells for retinal chemical communication the simulation has included both of these cells, enabling a demonstration of its capacity to simulate clusters containing heterogeneous glial cell types.

Fig. 6 and Fig. 7 of Newman (2001) plot the concentration profile of ATP and the wave radii of ATP and Ca^{2+} respectively. The plots detail the results of both the control experiment, where both extracellular and intercellular pathways are fully active, and experiments where the purinergic antagonist suramin (which competitively blocks ATP receptors) is applied. These results are for experiments performed on 'whole-mounted' retinas (see Newman (2001) for details).

7.1.1   Configuration

The physical structure of the astrocytes within the simulation was established by measurement of Fig. 7.1 from Newman (2001), which gave a radius of 5μm for soma and a distance between astrocyte centres of 40μm. Müller cells were measured from Newman (2001) as presenting a smaller (lateral) face than astrocytes and the population established from the experimental paper as well as from Distler et al. (1993) and Distler and Dreher (1996). Astrocytes were positioned in a regular grid pattern (see Fig. 7.1 and Fig. 7.2) and gap junctions were established between horizontally and vertically neighbouring astrocytes. Each astrocyte was surrounded by sixteen Müller cells to which they are connected by one-way (astrocyte to Müller cell) gap junctions (Zahs and Newman 1997). As Müller cells do not appear to be coupled in the retina (Newman 2001) there are no Müller cell to Müller cell gap junctions in the simulation.

7.1.2   Parameter values

Establishing an appropriate set of parameters for the simulation is not straightforward, as applying the parameters from existing theoretical models does not replicate the experimental data satisfactorily. This was expected, as there is large variability in glial cell characteristics such as permeability and chemical production rates (e.g. Lee et al. (1994)). Instead, theoretically derived parameters (see Table 3.1 for these parameters) were used as a starting point and adjusted as necessary to fit with the experimental results.

Control experiment simulation parameters

The principal resulting values for the control simulation were that for astrocytes the production rate of ATP (α_V) was reduced from $20,000\mu$Ms^{-1} to $10,000\mu$Ms^{-1}, the degradation rate of ATP (v_{deg}) was increased from 1s^{-1} to 8s^{-1} and the degradation of IP$_3$ (k_{deg}) was set to 0.10s^{-1} (the range of values in the literature for IP$_3$ degradation varies from 0.08s^{-1} in Höfer et al. (2002) to 1.25s^{-1} in Bennett et al. (2005) with a tendency to the lower value so values used within these simulations are well within the range of expected values for IP$_3$ degradation). Production rates for both IP$_3$ and ATP were significantly lower in Müller cells. Gap junction permeability (P_{ip3}) was set to $3\mu ms^{-1}$, the mean of the range given by Höfer et al. (2002), for astrocyte to astrocyte couplings and to $0.1\mu ms^{-1}$ for astrocyte to Müller cell coupling. The lower value for the latter coupling is based on the reduced importance of gap junctional coupling relative to extracellular communication reported in Newman (2001) for Müller cells. The saturation constant for IP$_3$ induced Ca^{2+} release (K_1) was increased from 0.03μM to 0.3μM (which slows the release of Ca^{2+}), this was necessary due to the relatively high IP$_3$ calculated by the simulations.

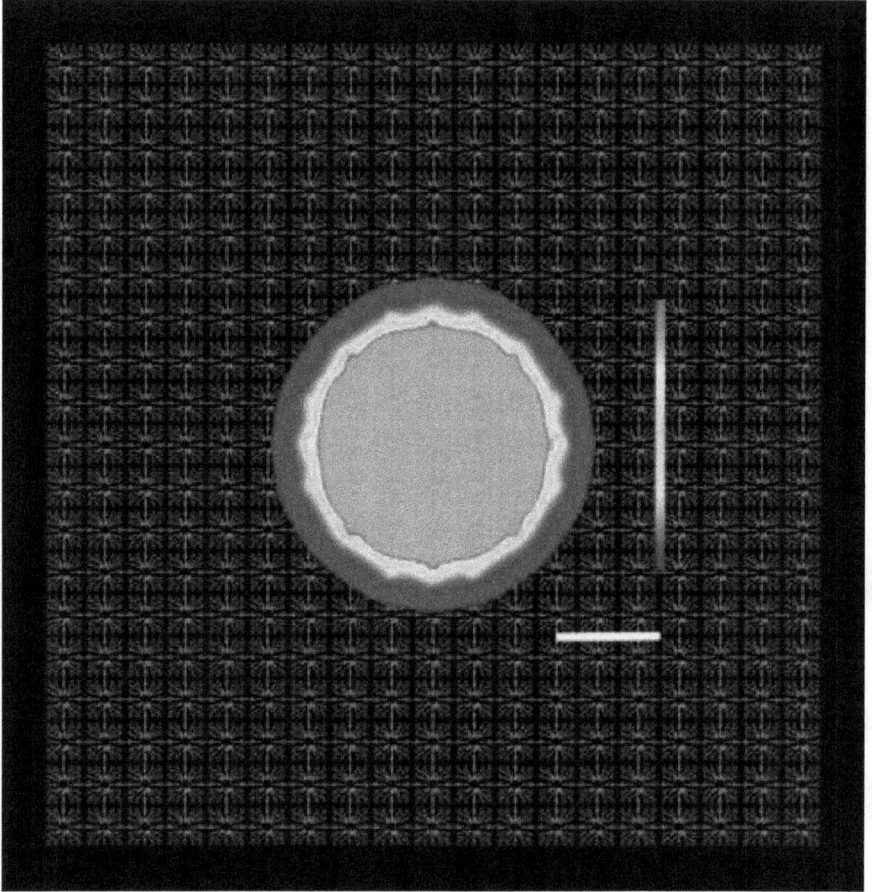

Figure 7.1: Structure of model for replication of Newman (2001). Astrocytes (the larger and less numerous cells) are arranged in a regular grid and are connected to their horizontal and vertical neighbours by gap junctions between processes. Müller cells (the smaller and more numerous cells) surround astrocytes in a square of sixteen cells and are connected by gap junctions to a single astrocyte only. There are a total of 6,137 cells in the whole simulation. The colouring represents ATP concentration. ATP release from the central cell is initiated with an external application of ATP and this image displays the results after 10 seconds. A close up view is supplied in Fig. 7.2. Scale bar, 100μm. Colour bar, 0μM - 3μM.

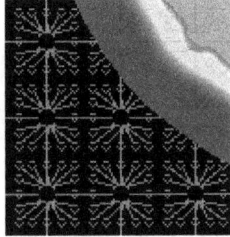

Figure 7.2: High resolution cropped view of Fig. 7.1, presented to provide a clear view of the structure of the simulation. Müller cells are arranged in a square around a central astrocyte and are connected via gap junctions to only that astrocyte. Each astrocyte itself is also connected to neighbouring astrocytes.

Suramin experiment simulation parameters

Suramin is a competitive puringergic receptor antagonist that should greatly reduce extracellular communication within a glial cluster. There were two parameter changes to the control definition used to replicate this.

- The activation rate (k_a) of G-protein was decreased from 0.017s^{-1} to 0.00017s^{-1}, which effectively mimics the expected effect of suramin.

- The next most important change made to the parameters was decreasing the initial release quantity by approximately $\frac{1}{3}$. This change was made in response to the experimental results, which could not be adequately fitted without this parameter modification (see discussion below). As the initial release in the experiment is provoked by mechanical stimulation on the outside cell well, near the puringergic receptors, it is possible that suramin does inhibit this initial release; however the entire release mechanism is currently poorly understood.

7.1.3   Results

Concentration profiles

Newman (2001) evaluated the concentration of ATP at various times using luciferin-luciferase bioluminescence and the results across a diameter of the retinal mount were plotted for both the control and suramin experiments on the whole-mounted retina. The experimental plots indicate that the application of suramin significantly decreases the peak concentration, radius and duration of the ATP waves. There appears to be some ambiguity in the results between Fig. 7 and Fig. 8 in Newman (2001); for instance the maximum wave radius for suramin is given as $30\mu m$ in

Fig. 7 however Fig. 6 indicates an ATP concentration $> 3\mu$M at a distance of 100μm after 6.6 seconds. Presumably this is due to data from different samples being used to plot the figures, which highlights the variability within clusters. Likewise, the asymmetric appearance of the plots in Fig. 6 of Newman (2001) suggest that the variation in individual astrocytes, as well as their position in the specimen, can have a strong influence on the resulting concentration profile (a result also predicted by the simulations).

The results from the simulation using the present model are given by Fig. 7.3. There is a good correlation between the two images with respect to peak concentrations, the shape of the time-courses of individual cells and the shape of the profile itself. The most significant deviation is in the more rapid decrease of ATP concentration in the centrally located cells of the simulation. This is primarily due to a modelled exhaustion of ATP stores (see Eq. 3.16) which appears to be necessary under the present model (see discussion below). If the rate of exhaustion is reduced then the simulations tend to maintain elevated concentrations of ATP indefinitely.

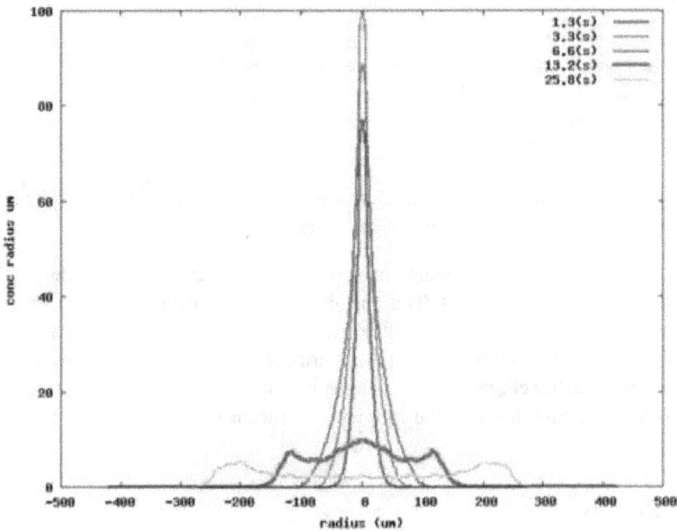

Figure 7.3: ATP concentration profiles at specified time steps for the control simulation (present model).

The ATP concentration profile from the suramin experiment of Newman (2001) is simulated in Fig. 7.4. When the parameters are adjusted to simulate the application of suramin there is, once again, good correlation between the plots with respect to peak concentrations and the pattern of time-courses, though the elevated concentration in the central cells again subsides to normal equilibrium concentrations rather earlier than displayed in the experimental results of Newman (2001).

When comparing the suramin simulation (Fig. 7.4) to the control simulation above (Fig. 7.3) it is readily apparent that the peak concentration in each cell is significantly smaller at each time step displayed. The radius of the wave is also significantly reduced as is the duration of the elevated ATP concentration. This conforms qualitatively to the differences between the experimental results and the experimental results.

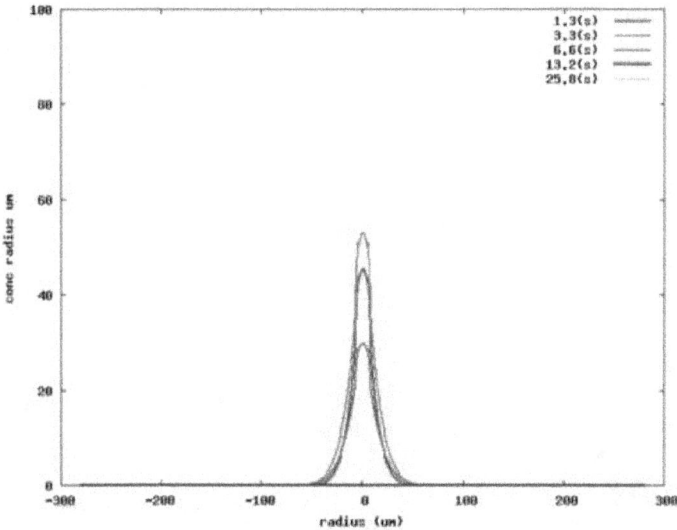

Figure 7.4: ATP concentration profile at selected time steps for the suramin experiment (present model).

Wave radius

The wave radius over the first 10 seconds of the experiment is displayed in Fig. 8 of Newman (2001). The wave radius of both ATP and Ca^{2+} is given (presumably the lack of a Ca^{2+} radius for suramin indicates that no significant increase in $[Ca^{2+}]$ was discerned) for both the control and suramin experiments. The comparison to the simulated results is given for control ATP (Fig. 7.5), control Ca^{2+} (Fig. 7.6) and suramin ATP (Fig. 7.7).

The most obvious difference between the control and suramin experimental plots is the significantly reduced radius and earlier peak radius in the suramin data. This difference is reflected in the simulation results, reinforcing the view that the reduced radius in suramin-affected specimens is due to the reduced activation of purinergic receptors and the inhibited initial release of ATP. The wave radii of the simulated and experimental results is similar in extent, though the simulation velocity does not decrease as rapidly as in the experimental results. It is possible that the regular morphology in the simulation encourages this, as it was observed that when gaps are introduced in the dense structure of the simulation it slows the wave spread.

The Ca^{2+} wave radius follows the ATP wave with a time-lag of around 2 seconds in the experimental results. This effect is visible in the simulation as well. It was observed that the duration of the lag was significantly influenced by the permeability of gap junctions, with lower permeabilities increasing the lag.

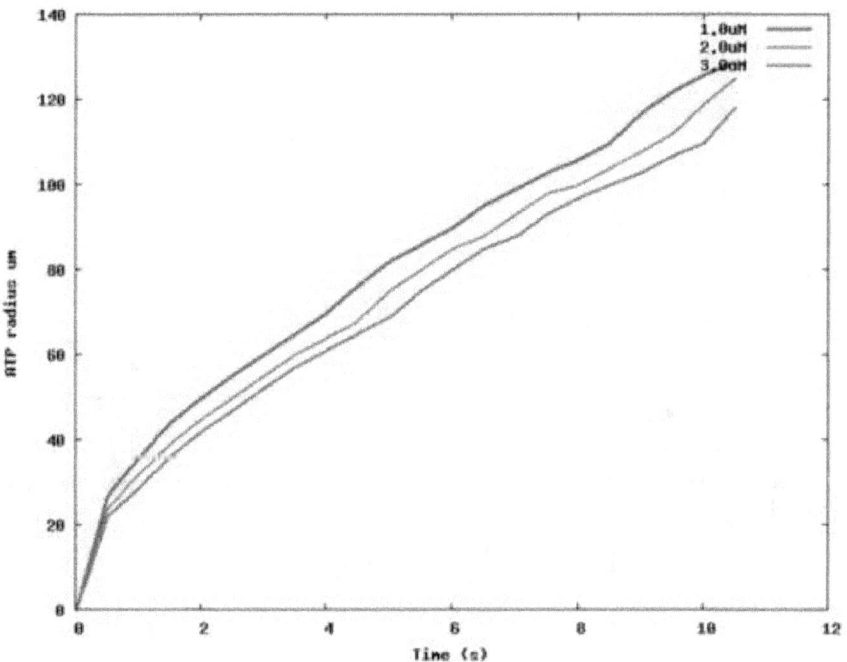

Figure 7.5: Calculated wave radius of ATP using the present model.

7.1.4 Discussion

The form of the initialisation was constrained by the experimental data. The experimental results peak after 4 seconds, which determines the start of the concentration decrease of the initialisation function in the simulation. The peak ATP concentration, particularly in the suramin experiment in which little regeneration is expected, determines the concentration that should be released over the

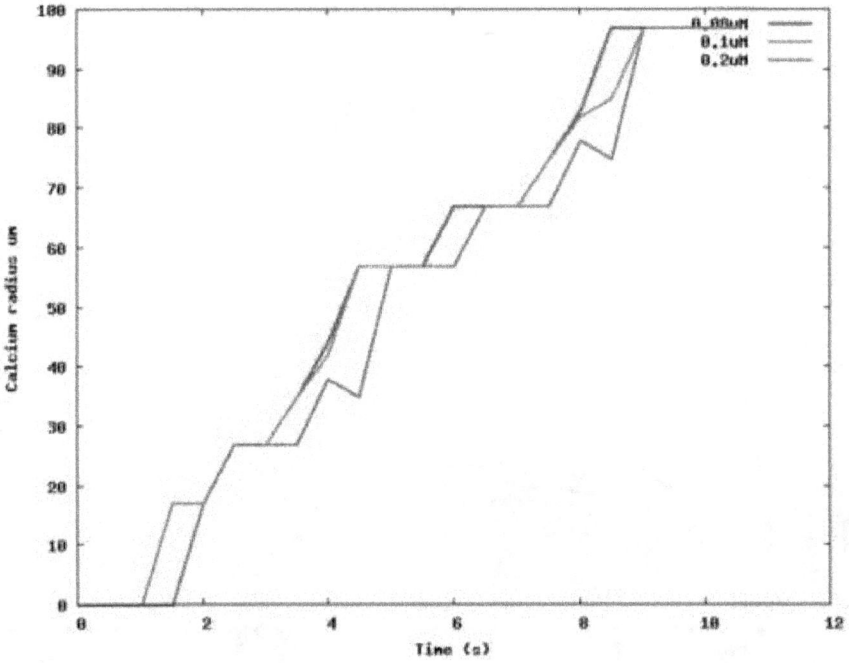

Figure 7.6: Calculated wave radius of Ca^{2+} from present model. There is a short lag visible in the radius when compared with Fig. 7.5. This corresponds to the time-lag observed in the results of Newman (2001).

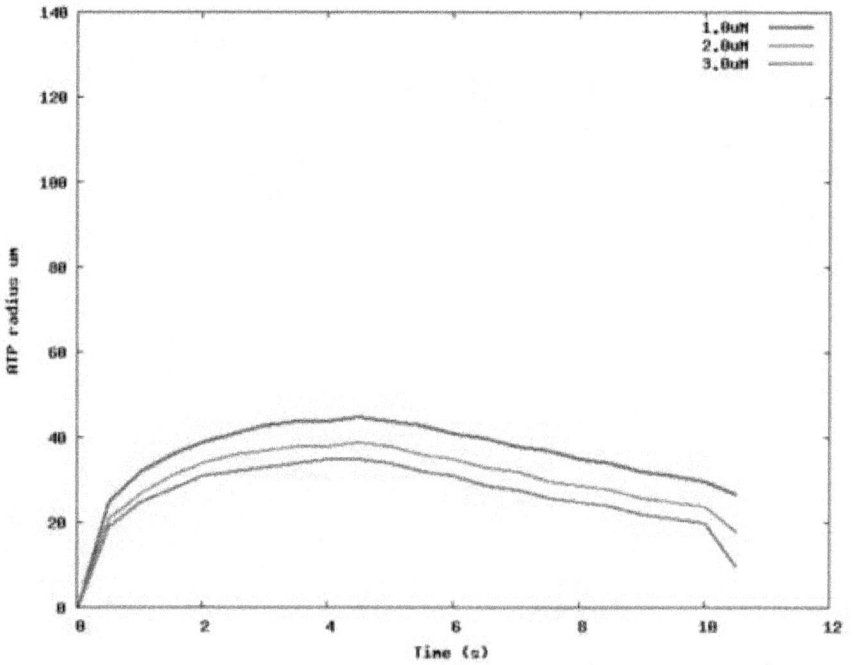

Figure 7.7: Calculated wave radius of ATP after application of suramin from present model.

first few seconds. Given a set of parameters determining characteristics such as ATP production together with the concentration at later times the initialising concentrations can be determined quite easily.

Determining the initialisation concentration using this process indicates that the initial release of ATP due to mechanical stimulation is quite high, with ATP concentrations above one molar per second being released from each point on the cell walls for the first few seconds. The experimental results show that the control has a peak concentration of around $90\mu M$ when a concentration of $3\mu M$ is sufficient to induce an intracellular Ca^{2+} wave. Using this information helped determine that the extracellular diffusion of ATP from the initial release dominates the peak concentrations early on in the time-courses. For the simulations reported here, the best fit to the experimental data required initialisation to occur over 10 seconds, with steeply decreasing release after 4 seconds. The ATP concentration for the first few seconds is determined principally by the diffusion of the initialising ATP and to a lesser extent the rate of ATP production from IP_3 (which is itself primarily influenced by the concentration of ATP at this time) and so when suramin is applied to the solution it is expected that the ATP concentration at these early times is almost solely due to the initial release caused by the mechanical stimulation (i.e. it does not involve much regeneration). The simulation demonstrated that to reach the required $50 - 90\mu M$ concentrations around $2,000 - 3,000\mu Ms^{-1}$ of ATP must be released from the stimulated cell for the first four seconds, subsequently decreasing to $750 - 1,500\mu Ms^{-1}$ by 10 seconds, after which time initialisation ceases. It should be noted that this surprisingly high release is due to the effects of diffusion which dissipates much of the concentration before it can build up to an excessive concentration. $3,000\mu Ms^{-1}$ is only $3\mu Mms^{-1}$, and combined with the effects of diffusion will not produce a concentration greater than $30\mu M$ without regeneration (see Fig. 7.8).

The 10 second duration for initialisation at the centre cell was unexpectedly long, however it was found to be the best fit for the experimental data after considering initial ATP bursts extending for as little as two seconds. Reviewing the literature shows that previous models, such as Sneyd et al. (1998), have used even longer durations for mechanically stimulated initialisations. Initialisation is assumed to occur via an externally provoked release of ATP rather than an elevation in mediator (e.g. IP_3) activity, this was chosen because elevating IP_3 to a sufficient concentration to release molar concentrations of ATP would require extremely high IP_3 concentrations in the present model.

Even with a conservative ATP diffusion coefficient of $200\mu m^2 s^{-1}$ (which is slower then the rate used in most theoretical papers), the concentration time-course of a pure diffusion (i.e. no regeneration) simulation given in Fig. 7.8 indicates that the furthest radius with which an initial release of $3,000\mu ms^{-1}$ over 4 seconds reaches the Ca^{2+} wave inducing threshold of $3\mu M$ is around $28\mu m$; similar to the experimental results for suramin, but too small for the control experiment, thereby demonstrating the role of regeneration in the formation of larger radius waves.

Whereas the ATP profile at earlier times and in more central cells is mainly determined by extracellular diffusion, at later times and in more radial cells the concentration, and particularly

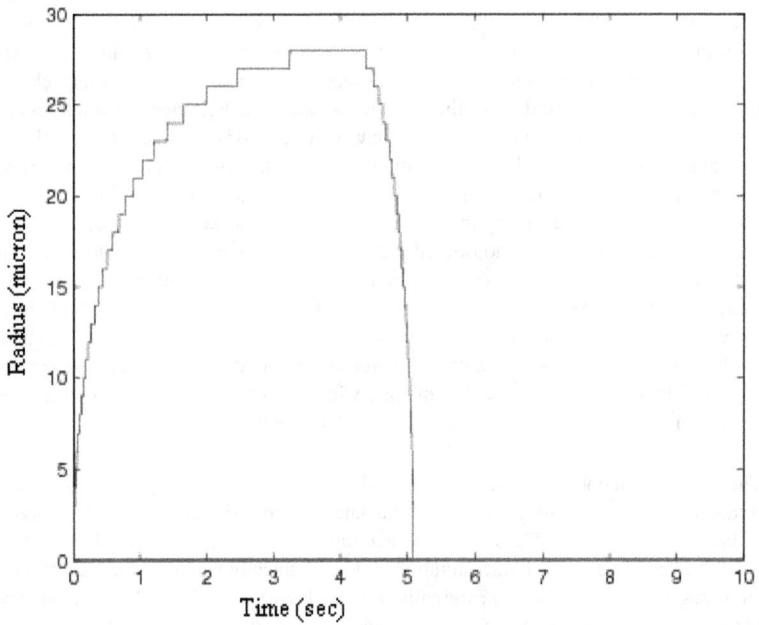

Figure 7.8: Wave radius for pure diffusion over a 2 dimensional grid with degradation. Threshold is 3μM and initialisation is $3,000\mu Ms^{-1}$ for 4 seconds. The reduction in the wave radius after initialisation ceases is rapid, demonstrating the need for regeneration to replicate the experiments reported in Newman (2001).

the radius, is much more influenced by the level of intercellular connectedness (i.e. number of processes and the permeability of the gap junctions) for the glia. It was found, in agreement with Höfer et al. (2002), that changes in the permeability of gap junctions could alter the wave spread from being finite to being infinite.

As noted above, the need for exhaustion of ATP stores affects the concentration in central cells at later times in the simulation. Without exhaustion, ATP concentrations in cells that exceed parameter-determined thresholds in chemical concentration will maintain an equilibrium state greater than that found the experimental results (see Appendix A). The problems this leads to in accurately replicating experimental results suggests that an alternate mechanism is employed biologically to inhibit uncontrolled growth of ATP – for example gap junctional release of ATP may slowly close the gap junctions, thereby reducing the ATP release over time.

Chapter 8

Discussion

8.1   Aims, Usage, Relevance and Critical Tests of the Model

The present model is intended to connect and extend previous models of chemical communication within glial cell clusters that simulate either gap junctional intercellular communication or puriner-gic receptor based extracellular communication. Many types of glial cells (Lee et al. 1994) use both methods and the present model is specifically targeted at allowing these cells to be simulated more accurately. In addition to the extension of previous models, the development of the present model is motivated by a need for a model implementation that produces fast simulations. Simple lane-ways of cells with neighbour to neighbour gap junctional connections execute in under five minutes and larger simulations consisting of hundreds of cells each with multiple gap junctionally connected processes execute in under an hour, even on relatively modest computer hardware. Included within the standard execution of the simulation are a range of graphical and numerical output files that provide detailed information on the concentration time-course, wave radius, concentration profile and other aspects of each of the chemicals involved.

The numerical implementation of the present model is executed by supplying a text definition file that contains the parameters and grid structure to be used for the simulation. It can be executed on any Java compliant platform (including Windows, Unix and Mac OS) and produces output in the form of comma separated data files and PNG graphics files. These data files provide concen-trations for each of the chemical species at each point in the grid for the specified time steps. The graphical output files provide easy to read displays of concentration time-courses, wave radius and concentration profiles.

While some glial cell communication is exclusively via intercellular gap junctions or exclu-sively via extracellular diffusion, it appears likely that many glial cells use both mechanisms to communicate within clusters. This biological fact underscores the relevance of the present model, the only model that incorporates regeneration in both mechanisms, to the field of theoretical models producing simulations of glial cell communication.

New discoveries that continue to expand the known role of glial cells in moderating cellular activity motivate the expansion of theoretical glial cell models, and the incorporation of the two primary communication mechanisms in astrocytes into the present model is a natural progression from previous models. The next evolution of these models will likely add neuronal communication along with other refinements as the various mechanisms modelled here are elucidated further.

Unlike some other theoretical models, the present model has been developed without the benefit of concurrent biological experimentation and so testing has been performed against previously published papers. In particular three theoretical papers (Sneyd et al. 1995, Höfer et al. 2002, Bennett et al. 2005) have been used to evaluate the present model's capacity for replicating intercellular and extracellular simulations individually, and one experimental paper (Newman 2001) has been used to evaluate its ability to replicate a cluster of glial cells utilising both mechanisms.

The three theoretical papers were each used to evaluate different capabilities of the present model. The replication of Sneyd et al. (1995) indicates that the present model can simulate intercellular non-regenerative passive diffusion scenarios in which a central IP_3 increase initiates a Ca^{2+} wave amongst neighbouring cells. The replication of Höfer et al. (2002) demonstrates a capacity to simulate intercellular waves that regenerate as a result of IP_3 and Ca^{2+} dynamics. The replicated simulation of preferential pathways as discussed in that paper further indicates the ability of the present model to study phenomena somewhat more intricate than chemical time-courses. The replication of Bennett et al. (2005) was included to demonstrate the capacity of the present model to simulate extracellular pathways utilising ATP as a messenger. The very close match to the results of the 3 dimensional scheme used in Bennett et al. (2005) supports the use of the 2 dimensional scheme utilised by the present model for reasons of performance.

8.2 Model

8.2.1 Equations

The model presented by this book is comprised of four principal equations that define the interactions between the four corresponding chemicals of interest. The production or release of each chemical is mediated as follows:

- G-protein is activated by the binding of ATP to purinergic receptors.

- IP_3 is produced by the activated G-protein and also by elevations in Ca^{2+} concentration.

- Intracellular Ca^{2+} release is mediated by increases in the concentration of IP_3.

• Extracellular ATP release is mediated by increases in the concentration of IP_3.

The equations of previous models have been used to derive the combined equations used here, however they have been modified where necessary with biologically justifiable changes.

G-protein. The G-protein equations are essentially the simplified forms of Lemon et al. (2003) used in Bennett et al. (2005). Within the present model the dissociation parameter has been split into two parameters, one of which represents the dissociation with the other representing additional variables such as the density of purinergic receptors.

Ca^{2+}. The Ca^{2+} equations are based on given by Fink et al. (1999) and as such are similar to the equations provided by Li and Rinzel (1994) which have become standard in models of this type. Independent pools for IP_3 or Ca^{2+} sensitive release of Ca^{2+} have been included in this model.

ATP. The ATP equations are based on those of Bennett et al. (2005). An extracellular degradation term has been included; it has a saturation equation form to represent the effect of ectonucleotidases. Bennett et al. (2005) include a χ term to their ATP production equation that represents the exhaustion of ATP stores. The present model extends this term to include a regenerative component.

IP_3. Both $PLC\beta$ and $PLC\delta$ production terms are included in the present model with the $PLC\beta$ terms being derived from Bennett et al. (2005) and $PLC\delta$ being derived from Höfer et al. (2002). IP_3 degradation is linear and intercellular flux is derived from Fick's law using a similar scheme to Höfer et al. (2002).

It should be noted that unlike the relatively well-defined equations governing Ca^{2+} dynamics, the equations that model ATP and IP_3 are conjectural adaptations of reaction-diffusion equations. G-protein dynamics have been modelled in a detailed way (Lemon et al. 2003); however the parameter values associated with the equations are not well-established. Until such time as these mechanisms are better understood there will be a lack of accuracy in models such as this. It is hoped that the present model may contribute to the development of understanding of these mechanisms.

The model is implemented numerically as a 2 dimensional grid. It was found through comparison with the 3 dimensional model presented in Bennett et al. (2005) (see Sec. 6.3) that this does not have a great impact on the results when a 2 dimensional arrangement of glial cells is used. Furthermore, while *in vitro* experiments are naturally 3 dimensional, they very often involve a 2 dimensional arrangement of glial cells in which imaging is also performed - and thus results collected - over a 2 dimensional layer at the surface of the experiment. A 2 dimensional arrangement is also appropriate in some *in vivo* simulations, such as those involving the retina (see Sec. 7.1).

8.2.2 Parameters

One of the purposes of a theoretical model is to predict values for unknown biological parameters, such as activation and deactivation rates, or the production and degradation rates for the concentrations of chemicals. Many of the parameters used in this model have been fitted to particular experiments or taken from biological experiments that do not necessarily relate to the CNS region of a particular simulation.

As can be seen from Table 3.1, there are potentially dozens of parameters used within a single simulation of which many will not have a strong certainty of accuracy. This diminishes the quantitative value of the predictions made by individual simulations.

The qualitative value of the simulations is less affected by this problem. Most of the parameter values are known to a reasonable accuracy and so the effect of changing particular aspects of the simulations gives insight into the effect that type of change (e.g. increase or decrease of production rates, greater variability in permeabilities etc) would have in biological experiments.

The present model also provides evidence for the value of parameters that are too difficult to determine experimentally. Such parameter values as the rate of IP_3 degradation and the rate of ATP production are within the range of previously theoretically established values while corresponding to experimental results and so help support the theoretically claimed parameter values. Likewise it is suggested that the dissociation constant for IP_3 induced Ca^{2+} production is higher in the retina than that in other CNS regions. The veracity of this claim will need to wait for advances in biological observation techniques.

8.2.3 Characteristics

The model equations and simulations have demonstrated the criteria that influence the establishment of diffusive, finitely regenerative or infinitely regenerative wave propagation within cell clusters. They relate to the dual stable nature of the ATP - IP_3 dynamics which supports the (theoretical) establishment of conditions within a glial cell in which the amount of release of ATP is sufficient to indefinitely regenerate the same concentration in subsequent releases. Höfer et al. (2002) demonstrated the mechanism which underlies this in intercellular waves and within this model it is demonstrated for extracellular waves. See Appendix A for a more detailed discussion of the mathematical basis of this characteristic.

Simulations using the present model indicate that the exhaustion of ATP stores, or the release induced desensitivity of ATP releasing receptors, is necessary to restore chemical concentrations to pre-existing equilibria. This prediction is naturally dependent on the form of the production and degradation equations, and is related to the situation described in the previous paragraph.

The present model has been used to evaluate the sensitivity of different criteria to different parameters. This can be accomplished using brute force techniques because of the reasonably fast execution time for simulations. For example, to determine the type of waves produced by different permeabilities and production rates in Sec. 6.2, a sequence of dozens of simulations was run in each of which the parameter values were changed slightly. Inspection of the results allowed determination of the resultant wave type.

Simulations using the present model exhibit different characteristics depending on the structure of the cell layout. Surprisingly small changes in the distance between cells can determine whether a wave is finitely or infinitely regenerative. The area of the glial cells has a similar influence on the wave type. It was found that this high sensitivity to the cell structure was greatly lessened when variability was introduced into the cellular properties. Simply having a ten percent variance in the ATP production rates between different cells was sufficient to reduce the sensitivity to positional changes. Similarly, while replicating the results of Höfer et al. (2002) (see Sec. 6.2), variations in gap junctional coupling strengths were found to induce the formation of preferential pathways. When the coupling strength was randomised it was found that, while different pathways were formed on each simulation, the ATP wave radius and velocity tended to be similar in each simulation. It appears likely that the variability in glial cells found in nature will tend to smooth out differences between behaviours in different clusters with similar 'average' properties.

Simulations run using the present model establish that the initialisation of the chemical concentration by external agents is generally the primary determinant of the wave radius and peak concentration. The duration and concentration of the initialisation is of such importance to the character of the subsequent wave in the simulations that the current lack of knowledge about the underlying biology of the initialisation limits the ability of theoretical models to make accurate predictions about the quantitative aspects of the glial wave. The need for further study on this subject is discussed below.

8.2.4   Future Experiments and Model Extension

Model extensions

The cooperative relationship between astrocytes and neurons through such mechanisms as glutamate signalling has lately become better understood (Hatton and Parpura 2004). There is as yet no published theoretical model describing this relationship. The present model, which already accommodates different glial cell types, could be expanded to included neuronal chemical reactions fairly simply. Modelling the electrical signalling within neurons, which operate on smaller timescale, is also achievable.

The morphologies of glial cells vary considerably. The present model assumes cells are circular, an approximation which prohibits the exploration of effects dependent on the actual shape of the cells. The simulations have demonstrated the importance of radius and position with the glial cells which suggests that the morphology of the glial cell, and in particular the variations in the morphologies of cells within a cluster, can have a dramatic effect on the resulting Ca^{2+} wave. With the addition of techniques for specifying arbitrary 2 dimensional morphologies these effects could be explored in detail.

Biological experiments

It became clear while performing simulations on the models utilising extracellular diffusion that the rate of degradation of ATP in the extracellular space is extremely important in determining the size the ATP wave, a phenomenon that makes intuitive sense. The literature gives many different values for ATP degradation (as discussed in Sec. 3.2.1); furthermore there is often ambiguity as to the rate of degradation of the produced ADP, AMP and adenosine, each of which may trigger responses in different types of purinergic receptors. It appears likely that there are vastly different degradation rates in different species and CNS regions; however, knowing the degradation rate in a given region would enable the single greatest improvement in the accuracy of simulations of extracellular ATP waves.

There are reports of conditions in which glial cells engage in excessive communication for indefinite periods of time (Wieseler-Frank and Watkins 2004). This appears to conform to the situation described in Appendix A where a higher equilibrium condition is established due to a combination of factors, for example a large burst of ATP or second-messenger or a change in key parameter values. Bennett et al. (2006) also found an apparently infinitely propagating ATP wave in a series of astrocytes *in vitro*, indicating that such a situation is biologically plausible. A potential experiment to test this condition would establish a circular lane-way of at least 1 mm radius containing regularly spaced astrocytes. After superfusion on the specimen is applied a wave would be initiated with a large concentration at a single point, producing either a finitely or infinitely propagating wave. If the wave is finite and terminates at around 1mm then that would indicate an exhaustion condition occurred at the initiated cell from which the cell had not recovered (Wang et al. (2000) demonstrate that a astrocyte may be temporarily depleted after stimulation), if the wave terminated before 1 mm then that would indicate that the astrocytes could not produce an infinite wave. An infinite wave, i.e. one which completes multiple revolutions of the circular lane-way, could have its concentration (at least of ATP and Ca^{2+}) measured to determine the higher equilibrium concentrations. Repeated experiments could elucidate the threshold of ATP that produces higher equilibrium states and the resultant infinite waves (see Fig. 8.1).

Greater elucidation of the agonist mechanism that results in the creation of a Ca^{2+} wave would be of great benefit. It is unknown which chemical is stimulated by the mechanism and it is unknown how long the effect lasts before regenerative effects become dominant. The simulations from the present model, and indeed from many preceding models, have made it clear how important the initial release is to the subsequent Ca^{2+} wave. Two experiments are suggested. To evaluate the agonist affected chemical a number of blockers and antagonists could be applied to an isolated cell

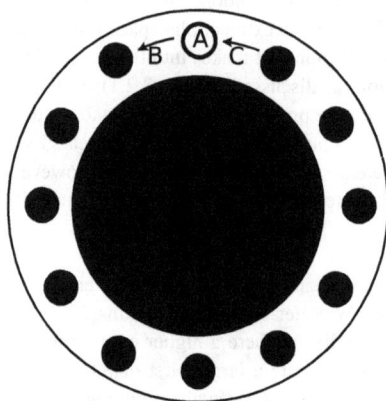

Figure 8.1: Proposed experiment to determine the maximum duration and radius of a glial calcium wave. Astrocytes are plated in a torus shaped area which is superfused to direct the extracellular diffusion in an anti-clockwise direction. The astrocyte denoted by (A) is stimulated causing it to release ATP in the direction of the arrow (B). If the wave reaches (C) then the astrocyte at (A) should have returned to its equilibrium concentration and will be excited again by the ATP. This potentially then leads to an indefinite propagation of the wave in repeated revolutions of the plate. If astrocytes can be demonstrated to propagate indefinitely then this may implicate them as candidates in long-term phenomena.

and then the cell would be stimulated. It would be expected that only those chemicals released as a direct response to the stimulation would increase in concentration. There are complications with this, not least of which is the lack of a marker for the candidate second messenger IP_3 (though the PIP_2 concentration could be determined). A second experiment to evaluate the duration of the initial release would also be of great benefit. By blocking the receptors that the initiating chemical binds to (assuming it can be identified) the duration of elevation of the concentration levels for the initiating chemical could be established. If degradation rates are known, and for some candidates such as IP_3 theoretical models have predicted degradation to a suitably narrow range, then the duration of release can be established.

8.3 Summary

The present model provides a set of equations that may be used to simulate the interaction of ATP, Ca^{2+}, G-protein and IP_3 to facilitate intercellular and extracellular communication between heterogeneous glial cells in 2 dimensions. The model defines interactions occurring both intracellularly, intercellularly and extracellularly.

The model has been numerically implemented in a computer program (Appendix B) with which simulation parameters may be easily defined using a text editor on a parameter file.

Simulations have been run to verify the accuracy of the model using existing papers, both experimental and theoretical. These simulations have demonstrated that the present model is able to replicate closely the results of existing theoretical papers and to simulate the results of more complex biological experiments.

Appendix A

Theoretical Analysis of Exhaustion and Elevated Equilibria

In vivo, propagating cellular waves are assumed to degenerate - that is they travel a finite distance and then dissipate to background concentrations. Some theoretical works (Bennett et al. 2005, Höfer et al. 2002) and, significantly, *in vitro* experimental work (Bennett et al. 2006) have suggested that in some cases these waves may, in theory, be infinitely regenerative.

Here the characteristics that determine whether a regenerative wave is finitely or infinitely regenerative are identified within a simple two-chemical model. The criteria as to whether a wave is finitely or infinitely regenerative is if the chemical concentration delivered from non-initiating upstream cells to downstream cells exceeds the lower bound of a basin of attraction to a higher concentration steady state that exists within each cell for the concentrations of the intracellular and extracellular chemical concentrations.

A simple model for regenerative waves involves an extracellularly diffusing chemical and an intracellular messenger chemical, each mediating the other chemical's release. One generic way to describe the dynamic concentration changes is:

$$\frac{\partial [E]}{\partial t} = D_E \nabla^2 [E] + \rho_E [I] - \gamma_E [E],$$

and

$$\frac{\partial [I]}{\partial t} = \rho_I [E] - \gamma_I [I], \tag{A.1}$$

where $[E]$ is the concentration of the extracellular diffusing chemical and $[I]$ is the concentration of the intracellular chemical. In the present model these would correspond to ATP and IP$_3$. Note that the extracellular concentration diffuses and that production of E occurs only at positions that are cell boundaries. This model fails to capture physiological processes accurately because any change in one concentration will, unless the parameter values are artificially balanced, lead to either unconstrained concentration increases or immediate decreases back to zero concentrations. By adding two extensions to this generic equation for the extracellular concentration more physiological behaviour can be described:

$$\frac{\partial [E]}{\partial t} = D_E \nabla^2 [E] + \rho_E \frac{([I] - [I]_{thres})}{[I] + K} - \gamma_E [E]. \tag{A.2}$$

The changes here describe a model where small changes in [I] do not lead to a change in [E] (concentrations below 0 are impossible) and the catalysts or receptors that enable the production or release of E can saturate. Both of these conditions are biologically justified.

The introduction of the threshold concentration provides a basin of attraction to a lower (normal) equilibrium state. The saturation equation provides an upper bound to [E], as $\lim_{[I] \to \infty} E = \frac{\rho_E}{\gamma_E}$.

This form of coupled PDEs permits upper and lower bounds (potential steady nodes) and a potentially unstable node (Fig. A.1). These attributes are integral to the formation of degenerative or infinite waves.

A1   Degenerative Formation

The formation of either infinite or degenerative waves is determined by the value of the unstable node and the corresponding basins of attraction for the stable nodes. Assuming a lane of evenly spaced homogeneous cells, if the contribution of [E] arriving from the production (not from the initialisation however) of E from upstream cells due to diffusion is greater than the value at the unstable node, the wave will propagate infinitely, since $[E]$ will reach $\frac{\rho_E}{\gamma_E}$ which is, by the assumption, a sufficient concentration to reach the next downstream cell with a concentration exceeding the unstable node value (Fig. A.2).

If the concentration arriving at downstream cells is less than the unstable node value, then the wave will terminate rapidly since the concentration will be attracted to the lower equilibrium value which is not sufficient to propagate a wave. At the very least, the concentration arriving at downstream cells will be monotonically less than that arriving at the previous cell. The rapidly terminating wave described can be considered diffusive rather than finitely regenerative, since the wave is never actively propagated, or is done so in only a very limited way (Fig. A.3).

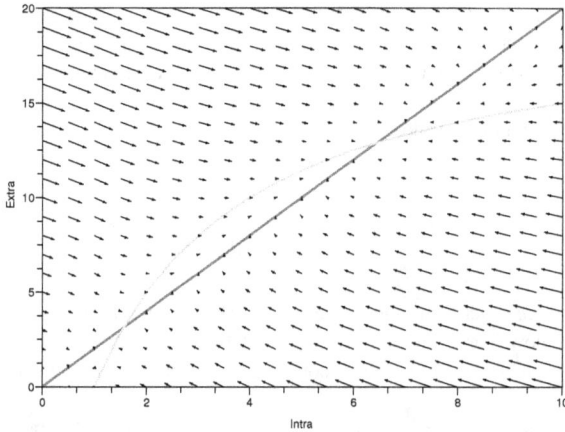

Figure A.1: Phase diagram and nullclines of the E-I system defined in Eq. A.1 and Eq. A.2. Nullclines are green and red. Note that there are two stable nodes and a single unstable node, typical of this form of coupled equations.

A middle scenario leads to finitely regenerative waves. Consider a lane of cells in which the concentration released from upstream cells is less, but close to, the unstable node value. Then consider that the initiating cell produces an extremely high concentration of E, considerably greater than the unstable node value. The addition of this initialising concentration as it diffuses to that produced by the excitation of cells (that themselves diffuse to only slightly less than the unstable node value) will lead to a [E] at all downstream cells within a radius determined by the diffusion of the initialisation to within the basin of attraction for the higher node. Hence a wave will form that has moderately decreasing, but greater than the unstable node value, concentrations of [E] for a certain distance, until a potentially rapid decrease in the wave to the lower stable node - at which point the wave has terminated. This type of wave can be described as finitely regenerative (Fig. A.4).

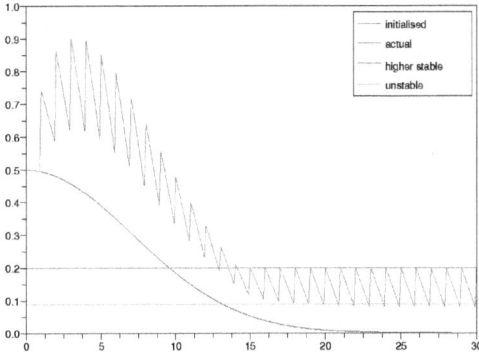

Figure A.2: Infinite Wave. The concentration of E arriving at each cell due to regeneration (i.e. excluding the initialising concentration) is always greater than u (the unstable node value). This produces an infinitely regenerating wave. Note that if the initial release is less than u then the infinite wave will not form.

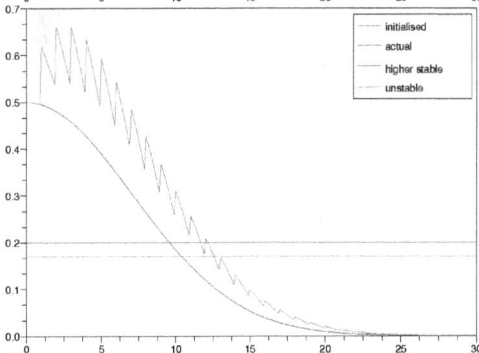

Figure A.3: Diffusive. The concentration of E arriving at each cell due to regeneration is less than u. The initialising concentration is insufficient to increase the concentration in any downstream cells to being above u, so the wave is essentially diffusive (though it is extended slightly by cellular production).

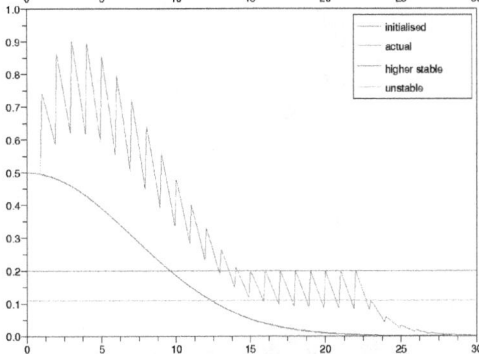

Figure A.4: Finite Wave. The concentration of E arriving at each cell due to regeneration is less than u. The addition of the initialising concentration increases the concentration to greater than u (and hence it then approaches the higher steady state) for a finite radius, but eventually the wave dissipates.

Figure A.5: Comparison of the three characteristic wave types. The wave is initialised from the left and travels towards the right. The y-axis gives the normalised concentration of extracellular chemical E and the x-axis shows the radius from the initialising source. 'Cells', where regeneration may occur, are located at each integer position. There are a number of parameters that when modified demonstrate each of these wave types; production rates, intercellular distance or the values of the stable and unstable nodes. In the cases above the value of the unstable node has been changed. Note that the plots here are simplified, for example cells are point sources and there is fast kinetics so that steady state concentrations are reached immediately.

A2   Determination of Nodes

A2.1   Nullclines

The I-nullcline exists when $\rho_I[E] = \gamma_I[I]$, hence

$$[I]_{null} = \frac{\rho_I}{\gamma_I}[E].\tag{A.3}$$

Considering that the steady state for the diffusive component of the equation within a degenerative wave with a free space boundary condition is 0, the E-nullcline exists when $\rho_E \frac{max(0,[I]-I_{thresh})}{[I]+K} = \gamma_E[E]$, hence

$$[E]_{null} = \frac{\rho_E}{\gamma_E} \frac{max(0,[I]-I_{thresh})}{[I]+K}.\tag{A.4}$$

A2.2   Critical Points

From the plots we expect three critical points: S_- (lower stable node) S_+ (higher stable node) and U, the unstable node. These points may change their character at various parameter values, though here we are principally interested in parameter values realistic to IP_3 mediated ATP waves.

S_- - The lower stable node

For $[I] \leq I_{thresh}$, $[E] = 0$ by Eq. A.4 which in turn implies that $[I] = 0$ by Eq. A.3. Hence (0,0) is a stable critical node, with a basin of attraction approximately around $[I] \leq I_{thresh}$.

The unstable and higher stable nodes

These nodes exist where $[I] > I_{thresh}$.

Using Eq. A.4:   The equation for a critical values for $[E]$ becomes:

$$[E]_{null} = \frac{\rho_E}{\gamma_E} \frac{\frac{\rho_I}{\gamma_I}[E]_{null} + K}{\frac{\rho_I}{\gamma_I}[E]_{null} - I_{thresh}}$$

or

$$\frac{\rho_I}{\gamma_I}[E]_{null}^2 - I_{thresh}[E]_{null} = \frac{\rho_E}{\gamma_E}(\frac{\rho_I}{\gamma_I}[E]_{null} + K)$$

so

$$\frac{\rho_I}{\gamma_I}[E]^2_{null} - (I_{thresh} + \alpha)[E]_{null} - \frac{\rho_E}{\gamma_E}K = 0$$

which has solutions given by

$$\frac{(I_{thresh} + \alpha) \pm \sqrt{(I_{thresh} + \alpha)^2 + 4\alpha K}}{2\frac{\rho_I}{\gamma_I}}.$$

Using [I]: The equation for a critical value of $[I]$ becomes:

$$[I] = \frac{\rho_I \rho_E}{\gamma_I \gamma_E} \frac{[I] - I_{thresh}}{[I] + K}$$

when substituting Eq. A.4 into Eq. A.3.

Let $\alpha = \frac{\rho_I \rho_E}{\gamma_I \gamma_E}$ hence

$$[I]^2 + [I]K = \alpha([I] - I_{thresh})$$

or

$$[I]^2 + (K - \alpha)[I] + \alpha I_{thresh} = 0$$

so the critical points are given by:

$$[I]_{s+} = \frac{(\alpha - K) + \sqrt{(K - \alpha)^2 - (4I_{thresh}\alpha)}}{2} \tag{A.5}$$

and

$$[I]_u = \frac{(\alpha - K) - \sqrt{(K - \alpha)^2 - (4I_{thresh}\alpha)}}{2}. \tag{A.6}$$

A2.3 Constraints On Critical Points

The parameters in the equations relate to biologically determined values and will all $\in (0, \infty)$. In some cases parameters like production rates may be zero, but these lead to trivial solutions. Assuming that there are no complex or negative solutions leads to two constraints:

constraint 1: no negative values

$$0 \leq 4I_{thresh}\alpha$$

which is only sensible as these parameters would be non-negative in any realistic situation; and

constraint 2: no complex solutions

$$4I_{thresh}\alpha < (K - \alpha)^2$$

which is not obvious, and indicates that the K and α parameters should not be too similar. Complex solutions are, however, not implausible biologically - oscillatory behaviour has been observed for intracellular Ca^{2+} waves in glial cells - though they are not known to occur for extracellular waves.

A3 Stability

The Jacobian from Eq. A.3 and Eq. A.4 is:

$$J = \begin{pmatrix} \gamma_I & \rho_E \\ \rho_E \frac{K+I_{thresh}}{(I+K)^2} & -\gamma_E \end{pmatrix}.$$

Hence, for $[I]_{crit}$, the trace and determinant are:

$$\tau = -(\gamma_I + \gamma_E)$$

$$\Delta = \gamma_I\gamma_E - \rho_E^2(K + I_{thresh})(\frac{(\alpha - K) \pm \sqrt{(K - \alpha)^2 - (4I_{thresh}\alpha}}{2} + K)^{-2}.$$

For realistic parameter values the discriminant may be approximated to:

$$\Delta_+^* = \gamma_I\gamma_E(1 - \frac{\gamma_I\gamma_E K}{\rho_I^2})$$

and

$$\Delta_-^* = \gamma_I\gamma_E - \frac{\rho_E^2}{K}.$$

Thus for all positive (and hence realistic) degradation values, $\tau \in (-\infty, 0)$ giving stable nodes for $\Delta > 0$ and saddle nodes for $\Delta < 0$. For typical parameter values used in this model (Table 3.1), $\Delta_-^* < 0$ and $\Delta_+^* > 0$. Stable spiral can occur for Δ_+^*, very high K or very low ρ_I values are required.

A4 Implications

Applying standard parameter values for IP_3 and ATP to the non-zero critical point formulae produce the two critical points, a saddle node which is near zero and a stable node that is much higher than any reasonable concentration. The basin of stability for the (much) higher valued stable node starts at very low values of $[I]$ and $[E]$.

The low concentrations for the unstable node, significantly lower than concentrations used to mark wave edges, introduce a problem in that for a wave to form the concentrations required will tend toward (physically implausible) concentrations as their steady state. For the concentrations to tend back down to the lower stable node an additional mechanism is required. The most likely are either exhaustion of cellular stores or slow-acting inhibitory receptors. These are represented in the present model by Eq. 3.16.

A4. IMPLICATIONS

Appendix B

Computer Implementation Source Code

The source code is freely available by emailing the author at jedwards@maths.usyd.edu.au

Bibliography

Allbritton NL, Meyer T and Stryer L 1992 Range of messenger action of calcium ion and inositol 1, 4, 5-trisphosphate *Science* **258**(5089), 1812.

Anderson CM and Swanson RA 2000 Astrocyte glutamate transport: review of properties, regulation, and physiological functions *Glia* **32**(1), 1–14.

Armstrong RC 2000 'Immunofluorescent imaging of astrocyte'.
URL: *http://upload.wikimedia.org/wikipedia/en/c/cd/Gfapastr5.jpg*

Atri A, Amundson J, Clapham D and Sneyd J 1993 A single-pool model for intracellular calcium oscillations and waves in the Xenopus laevis oocyte *Biophysical Journal* **65**(4), 1727–1739.

Batter DK, Corpina RA, Roy C, Spray DC, Hertzberg EL and Kessler JA 1992 Heterogeneity in gap junction expression in astrocytes cultured from different brain regions *Glia* **6**(3), 213–221.

Bellinger S 2005 Modeling calcium wave oscillations in astrocytes *Neurocomputing* **65**, 843–850.

Bennett MR, Buljan V, Farnell L and Gibson WG 2006 Purinergic junctional transmission and propagation of calcium waves in spinal cord astrocyte networks *Biophysical Journal* **91**(9), 3560.

Bennett MR, Farnell L and Gibson WG 2005 A quantitative model of purinergic junctional transmission of calcium waves in astrocyte networks *Biophysical Journal* **89**(4), 2235–2250.

Bennett MV, Barrio LC, Bargiello TA, Spray DC, Hertzberg E and Saez JC 1991 Gap junctions: new tools, new answers, new questions *Neuron* **6**(3), 305–320.

Berridge MJ, Bootman MD and Lipp P 1998 Calcium–a life and death signal *Nature* **395**(6703), 645–648.

Bushong EA, Martone ME, Jones YZ and Ellisman MH 2002 Protoplasmic astrocytes in CA1 stratum radiatum occupy separate anatomical domains *Journal of Neuroscience* **22**(1), 183–192.

Butt AM and Ransom BR 1993 Morphology of astrocytes and oligodendrocytes during development in the intact rat optic nerve *The Journal Of Comparative Neurology* **338141**, 158.

Charles A 1998 Intercellular calcium waves in glia *Glia* **24**(1), 39–49.

Coco S, Calegari F, Pravettoni E, Pozzi D, Taverna E, Rosa P, Matteoli M and Verderio C 2003 Storage and release of ATP from astrocytes in culture *Journal of Biological Chemistry* **278**(2), 1354–1362.

Cornell-Bell AH, Finkbeiner SM, Cooper MS and Smith SJ 1990 Glutamate induces calcium waves in cultured astrocytes: long-range glial signaling *Science* **247**(4941), 470.

Cotrina ML, Lin JHC, Alves-Rodrigues A, Liu S, Li J, Azmi-Ghadimi H, Kang J, Naus CCG and Nedergaard M 1998 Connexins regulate calcium signaling by controlling ATP release *Proceedings of the National Academy of Sciences* **95**(26), 15735–15740.

De Young GW and Keizer J 1992 A single pool IP 3-receptor based model for agonist stimulated Ca 2+ oscillations *Proceedings of the National Academy of Sciences* **89**, 9895–9899.

Distler C and Dreher Z 1996 Glia cells of the monkey retina-II. Muller cells *Vision Research* **36**(16), 2381–2394.

Distler C, Weigel H and Hoffmann KP 1993 Glia cells of the monkey retina-I. Astrocytes *The Journal of Comparative Neurology* **333**(1), 134–147.

Dunwiddie TV, Diao L and Proctor WR 1997 Adenine nucleotides undergo rapid, quantitative conversion to adenosine in the extracellular space in rat hippocampus *Journal of Neuroscience* **17**(20), 7673–7682.

Dupont G, Berridge MJ and Goldbeter A 1991 Signal-induced Ca2+ oscillations: properties of a model based on Ca (2+)-induced Ca2+ release *Cell Calcium* **12**(2-3), 73–85.

Eberhard M and Erne P 1991 Calcium binding to fluorescent calcium indicators: calcium green, calcium orange and calcium crimson *Biochemical and biophysical research communications* **180**(1), 209–215.

Fink CC, Slepchenko B and Loew LM 1999 Determination of time-dependent inositol-1, 4, 5-trisphosphate concentrations during calcium release in a smooth muscle cell *Biophysical Journal* **77**(1), 617–628.

Gallagher CJ and Salter MW 2003 Differential properties of astrocyte calcium waves mediated by P2Y1 and P2Y2 receptors *Journal of Neuroscience* **23**(17), 6728–6739.

Gilkey JC, Jaffe LF, Ridgway EB and Reynolds GT 1978 A free calcium wave traverses the activating egg of the medaka, Oryzias latipes *The Journal of Cell Biology* **76**(2), 448–466.

Gosling J 2000 *The Java language specification* Addison-Wesley.

Guthrie PB, Knappenberger J, Segal M, Bennett MVL, Charles AC and Kater SB 1999 ATP released from astrocytes mediates glial calcium waves *Journal of Neuroscience* **19**(2), 520–528.

Hassinger TD, Guthrie PB, Atkinson PB and Bennett M 1996 An extracellular component in propagation of astrocytic calcium waves *Procedings of the National Academy of Sciences* **93**, 13268–13273.

Hatton GI and Parpura V 2004 *Glial neuronal signaling* Springer.

Haustein S 2005 kXML Project Technical report visited 05-01-01. http://www. kxml. org.

Haydon PG 2001 Glia: listening and talking to the synapse *Nature Reviews Neuroscience* **2**(3), 185–193.

Höfer T, Venance L and Giaume C 2002 Control and plasticity of intercellular calcium waves in astrocytes: A modeling approach *Journal of Neuroscience* **22**(12), 4850–4859.

Holopainen I, Enkvist MO and Akerman KE 1989 Glutamate receptor agonists increase intracellular Ca2+ independently of voltage-gated Ca2+ channels in rat cerebellar granule cells *Neuroscience Letters* **98**(1), 57–62.

Hubley MJ, Locke BR and Moerland TS 1996 The effects of temperature, pH, and magnesium on the diffusion coefficient of ATP in solutions of physiological ionic strength *Biochimica et biophysica acta* **1291**(2), 115–121.

Iacobas DA, Suadicani SO, Spray DC and Scemes E 2006 A stochastic two-dimensional model of intercellular Ca2+ wave spread in glia *Biophysical Journal* **90**(1), 24–41.

Keener JP, Wiggins S, Sirovich L, Kadanoff LP and Sneyd J 2001 *Mathematical Physiology* Springer.

Kettenmann H and Ransom BR 2005 *Neuroglia* Oxford University Press.

Kimelberg HK, Goderie SK, Higman S, Pang S and Waniewski RA 1990 Swelling-induced release of glutamate, aspartate, and taurine from astrocyte cultures *Journal of Neuroscience* **10**(5), 1583–1591.

Kupferman R, Mitra PP, Hohenberg PC and Wang SS 1997 Analytical calculation of intracellular calcium wave characteristics *Biophysical Journal* **72**(6), 2430–2444.

Lazarowski ER, Homolya L, Boucher RC and Harden TK 1997 Identification of an ecto-nucleoside diphosphokinase and its contribution to interconversion of P2 receptor agonists *Journal of Biological Chemistry* **272**(33), 20402–20407.

L'Ecuyer P, Meliani L and Vaucher J 2002 SSJ: a framework for stochastic simulation in Java *Proceedings of the 34th conference on Winter simulation: exploring new frontiers* **1**, 234–242.

Lee SH, Kim WT, Cornell-Bell AH and Sontheimer H 1994 Astrocytes exhibit regional specificity in gap-junction coupling *Glia* **11**(4), 315–325.

Lemon G, Gibson WG and Bennett MR 2003 Metabotropic receptor activation, desensitization and sequestration-I: modelling calcium and inositol 1, 4, 5-trisphosphate dynamics following receptor activation *Journal of Theoretical Biology* **223**(1), 93–111.

Leybaert L, Paemeleire K, Strahonja A and Sanderson MJ 1998 Inositol-trisphosphate-dependent intercellular calcium signaling in and between astrocytes and endothelial cells *Glia* **24**(4), 398–407.

Li YX and Rinzel J 1994 Equations for InsP3 receptor-mediated [Ca2+] oscillations derived from a detailed kinetic model: a Hodgkin-Huxley like formalism *Journal Theoretical Biology* **166**(4), 461–473.

Lytton J, Westlin M, Burk SE, Shull GE and MacLennan DH 1992 Functional comparisons between isoforms of the sarcoplasmic or endoplasmic reticulum family of calcium pumps *Journal of Biological Chemistry* **267**(20), 14483–14489.

Mahama PA and Linderman JJ 1994 A Monte Carlo study of the dynamics of G-protein activation *Biophysical Journal* **67**(3), 1345–1357.

Martins-Ferreira H, Nedergaard M and Nicholson C 2000 Perspectives on spreading depression *Brain Research Reviews* **32**(1), 215–234.

Miyawaki A, Llopis J, Heim R, McCaffery JM, Adams JA, Ikura M and Tsien RY 1997 Fluorescent indicators for Ca2+ based on green fluorescent proteins and calmodulin *Nature* **388**(6645), 882–887.

Nagy JI and Rash JE 2003 Astrocyte and oligodendrocyte connexins of the glial syncytium in relation to astrocyte anatomical domains and spatial buffering *Cell Communication & Adhesion* **10**(4), 401–406.

Newman EA 2001 Propagation of intercellular calcium waves in retinal astrocytes and Müller cells *Journal of Neuroscience* **21**(7), 2215–2223.

Newman EA and Zahs KR 1997 Calcium waves in retinal glial cells *Science* **275**(5301), 844–847.

Osipchuk Y and Cahalan M 1992 Cell-to-cell spread of calcium signals mediated by ATP receptors in mast cells *Nature* **359**, 241–244.

Pasti L, Volterra A, Pozzan T and Carmignoto G 1997 Intracellular calcium oscillations in astrocytes: a highly plastic, bidirectional form of communication between neurons and astrocytes in situ *Journal of Neuroscience* **17**(20), 7817–7830.

Perea G and Araque A 2005 Synaptic regulation of the astrocyte calcium signal *Journal of Neural Transmission* **112**(1), 127–135.

Peters A, Palay SL and Webster H 1991 *The fine structure of the nervous system: neurons and their supporting cells* Oxford University Press.

Pugh EN and Lamb TD 2000 *Handbook of Biological Physics* Elsevier Science BV Amsterdam.

Queiroz G, Meyer DK, Meyer A, Starke K and von Kugelgen I 1999 A study of the mechanism of the release of ATP from rat cortical astroglial cells evoked by activation of glutamate receptors *Neuroscience* **91**(3), 1171–1181.

Ramon y Cajal S 1909 *Histology of the nervous system of man and vertebrates* Oxford University Press.

Ransom BR and Ye ZC 2005 *Gap Junctions and hemichannels* Oxford University Press.

Rash JE, Yasumura T, Davidson KG, Furman CS, Dudek FE and Nagy JI 2001 Identification of cells expressing Cx43, Cx30, Cx26, Cx32 and Cx36 in gap junctions of rat brain and spinal cord *Cell Communication and Adhesion* **8**(4-6), 315–320.

Ridgway EB, Gilkey JC and Jaffe LF 1977 Free calcium increases explosively in activating medaka eggs *Proceedings of the National Academy of Sciences* **74**(2), 623–627.

Salter MW and Hicks JL 1995 Atp causes release of intracellular ca2+ via the phopholipase c beta/ip3 pathway in astrocytes from the dorsal spinal cord *Journal of Neuroscience* **15**(4), 2961–2971.

Savchenko VL, McKanna JA, Nikonenko IR and Skibo GG 2000 Microglia and astrocytes in the adult rat brain: comparative immunocytochemical analysis demonstrates the efficacy of lipocortin 1 immunoreactivity *Neuroscience* **96**(1), 195–203.

Sneyd J, Wetton BT, Charles AC and Sanderson MJ 1995 Intercellular calcium waves mediated by diffusion of inositol trisphosphate: a two-dimensional model *American Journal of Physiology - Cell Physiology* **268**(6), 1537–1545.

Sneyd J, Wilkins M, Strahonja A and Sanderson MJ 1998 Calcium waves and oscillations driven by an intercellular gradient of inositol (1, 4, 5)-trisphosphate *Biophysical Chemistry* **72**, 101–109.

Stamatakis M. and Mantzaris NV 2006 Modeling of ATP-mediated signal transduction and wave propagation in astrocytic cellular networks *Journal of Theoretical Biology* **241**, 649–668.

Stout CE, Costantin JL, Naus CCG and Charles AC 2002 Intercellular calcium signaling in astrocytes via ATP release through connexin hemichannels *Journal of Biological Chemistry* **277**(12), 10482–10488.

Taylor CW and Putney JW 1985 Size of the inositol 1, 4, 5-trisphosphate-sensitive calcium pool in guinea-pig hepatocytes *Biochemical Journal* **232**, 435–438.

Venance L, Stella N, Glowinski J and Giaume C 1997 Mechanism involved in initiation and propagation of receptor-induced intercellular calcium signaling in cultured rat astrocytes *Journal of Neuroscience* **17**(6), 1981–1992.

Verselis V, White RL, Spray DC and Bennett MV 1986 Gap junctional conductance and permeability are linearly related *Science* **234**(4775), 461.

Volterra A, Magistretti PJ and Haydon PG 2002 *Intercellular calcium waves in astrocytes: underlying mechanisms and functional significance* Oxford University Press.

Volterra A and Meldolesi J 2005 Astrocytes, from brain glue to communication elements: the revolution continues *Nature Reviews Neuroscience* **6**(8), 626–640.

Wang Z, Haydon PG and Yeung ES 2000 Direct observation of calcium-independent intercellular ATP signaling in astrocytes *Analytical Chemistry* **72**(9), 2001–7.

Wieseler-Frank, J Maier SF and Watkins LR 2004 Glial activation and pathological pain *Neurochemistry International* **45**(2-3), 389–395.

Wu D and Mori N 1999 Extracellular ATP-induced inward current in isolated epithelial cells of the endolymphatic sac *Biochimica Et Biophysica Acta* **1419**(1), 33–42.

Xu T, Naraghi M, Kang H and Neher E 1997 Kinetic studies of Ca2+ binding and Ca2+ clearance in the cytosol of adrenal chromaffin cells *Biophysical Journal* **73**(1), 532–545.

Zahs KR and Newman EA 1997 Asymmetric gap junctional coupling between glial cells in the rat retina *Glia* **20**(1), 10–22.

Ziganshin AU, Hoyle CHV and Burnstock G 1994 Ecto-enzymes and metabolism of extracellular ATP *Drug Development Research* **32**(3), 134–146.

Ziganshin AU, Ziganshina LE, King BF and Burnstock G 1996 Differential degradation of extracellular adenine nucleotides by folliculated oocytes of Xenopus laevis *Comparative Biochemistry and Physiology Part A: Physiology* **114**(4), 335–340.

www.ingramcontent.com/pod-product-compliance
Lightning Source LLC
Chambersburg PA
CBHW061609220326
41598CB00024BC/3504